THE HIDDEN SUGAR TRAP (T2)

Master the science, Break-free from myths, and reclaim your health for life

Dr. Vicki Loftin

Table of Contents

INTRODUCTION

1.1 What is diabetes type 2?

Type 2 diabetes, a chronic metabolic disease, is characterized by elevated blood sugar levels caused by insulin resistance and decreased insulin synthesis. Genetics and lifestyle factors primarily cause Type 2 diabetes, while the body's immune system attacks insulin-producing cells in Type 1 diabetes. It accounts for 90–95% of all cases of diabetes worldwide, making it the most prevalent form of the disease.

Comprehensive Blood Sugar and Insulin Regulation

Understanding how insulin functions in the body is critcal to understanding what type 2 diabetes entails. The pancreas, and especially the beta cells in the islets of Langerhans, produce the hormone insulin. Controlling blood sugar (glucose) levels is its main duty. Your digestive system converts carbs into glucose when you consume them, which then enters your circulation. In reaction, the pancreas produces insulin, which facilitates the body's cells' absorption of glucose for immediate use as energy or storage.

This procedure is precisely calibrated for a healthy person, guaranteeing that blood sugar levels stay within a restricted, healthy range. But in a person with type 2 diabetes, this mechanism breaks down. The body's cells become less responsive to insulin as a result of their increased resistance to its effects. As a result, the pancreas produces more insulin, but eventually it is unable to meet the body's needs. This results in hyperglycemia, a condition in which there is an excess of glucose in the blood.

Significance and Prognosis

Many patients with type 2 diabetes may not have been aware of their condition for years since it frequently develops gradually. Because of its delayed start and potential for difficult early identification, routine screening is essential, particularly for those who are more vulnerable. The following are typical signs of type 2 diabetes:

Repeated urination: Urine is the body's attempt to flush off extra glucose.

Increased thirst: Recurrent urination may cause dehydration, which makes thirst last longer.

Fatigue: The body may feel exhausted all the time because glucose isn't getting into the cells to be utilized as fuel.

Disturbed vision: Elevated blood sugar levels might cause fluid to be drawn out of the eye's lenses, impairing vision.

Slow healing wounds: Hyperglycemia may affect the immune system and blood flow, which can delay the healing of wounds.

Unexplained weight loss: While Type 1 diabetes is more common, some Type 2 diabetics may lose weight as a result of their bodies' improper use of glucose.

Usually, many blood tests are required to confirm the diagnosis of type 2 diabetes. The most typical ones are as follows:

Fasting Blood Glucose Test: After an overnight fast, blood sugar is measured. Diabetes is indicated by a test result of 126 mg/dL or above on two different occasions.

A1C Test: Indicates the average blood sugar levels throughout the previous two to three months. A diagnosis of diabetes is made at a level of 6.5% or above.

Oral Glucose Tolerance Test (OGTT): This test gauges blood sugar levels both before and after consuming a beverage that contains glucose. After two hours, a reading of 200 mg/dL or above suggests diabetes.

Dangers Factors

Type 2 diabetes is a result of several variables, which include:

Genetics: An important factor is family history. Your risk increases if you have a parent or sibling with type 2 diabetes.

Age: Although type 2 diabetes may strike anybody at any age, beyond the age of 45, the risk rises.

Obesity: Since it aggravates insulin resistance, excess body fat, especially around the belly, is a major risk factor.

Physical Inactivity: Type 2 diabetes is strongly associated with a lack of consistent exercise.

Ethnicity: People from certain ethnic backgrounds, including Native Americans, Asian Americans, African Americans, and Hispanics, are more vulnerable.

Diet: The risk of type 2 diabetes is increased by a diet heavy in processed foods, bad fats, and refined sugars.

The Diabetes Type 2 Progression

Diabetes type 2 is often characterized as a disorder that progresses. Lifestyle changes, such as losing weight, eating better, and exercising more, may significantly lower blood sugar levels in the early stages. Nevertheless, when the illness worsens, these interventions may not be as successful, and medication or insulin treatment could be necessary to keep blood sugar under control.

Serious consequences such as cardiovascular disease, nerve damage (neuropathy), kidney illness (nephropathy), eye damage (retinopathy), and foot issues may arise from uncontrolled diabetes over time. The harmful effects of persistently elevated blood sugar on blood vessels and neurons are the cause of these problems.

1.2 A Historical Overview

Gaining insight into the historical background of type 2 diabetes will help us better understand how the illness has progressed in terms of both diagnosis and treatment.

Comprehensive knowledge of diabetes

Diabetes has been understood for thousands of years. The oldest accounts date back to 1500 BCE, when doctors in ancient Egypt reported a disease marked by frequent urination. This is documented in one of the earliest medical records, the Ebers Papyrus. The Greek word "siphon," which describes the disease's frequent urination, is where the name "diabetes" originates.

An illness known as "Madhumeha" (honey urine) was discovered by Indian doctors in antiquity. Affected people's sweet-smelling urine drew ants to them. This was one of the first observations linking diabetes to sugar metabolism.

The Discovery of Sugar in Urine Throughout the Middle Ages

European doctors like Avicenna (Ibn Sina) continued to record diabetes throughout the Middle Ages. They identified two types of the illness: type 1 diabetes, which is more prevalent in younger people, and type 2 diabetes, which is more frequent in older people. But until the 17th century, when English physician Thomas Willis discovered that certain diabetes patients' urine had a sweet taste, suggesting the presence of sugar, the precise nature of the illness remained unknown.

19th and 20th Centuries: Knowledge Progression
Significant progress was made in our knowledge of diabetes throughout the 19th century. These discoveries opened the door for more studies into the role of the pancreas in diabetes. In 1815, French chemist Michel Eugène Chevreul confirmed that sugar was present in diabetic urine. In 1848, German physician Paul Langerhans identified the cell clusters in the pancreas that would later be named "islets of Langerhans."

The first direct evidence connecting the pancreas to diabetes was found in 1889, when German researchers Joseph von Mering and Oskar Minkowski removed the pancreas from dogs and saw that the animals developed severe diabetes.

The 1921 discovery of insulin by Canadian scientists Frederick Banting and Charles Best marked the beginning of the 20th century. Insulin provided a life-saving medicine that transformed the treatment of diabetes, especially type 1 diabetes. It also emphasized the distinctions between Type 1 and Type 2 diabetes since not all individuals with diabetes need insulin.

The Contemporary Age: Acknowledging Type 2 Diabetes as a Worldwide Health Concern: Type 2 diabetes became more common as the 20th century went on, especially in developed countries. This rise was strongly associated with lifestyle changes, such as increased sedentary activity and diets high in processed foods and sweets. Type 2 diabetes had grown to be a significant public health issue by the late 20th century.

In 1980, the World Health Organization (WHO) started tracking the incidence of diabetes globally after realizing the disease was becoming more widespread. Additionally, the importance of obesity as a significant risk factor became increasingly apparent, which increased the focus on preventative efforts.

New Type 2 diabetes treatment options were made possible by the mid-20th century introduction of oral hypoglycemic medications. Many people were able to achieve improved blood sugar control without the need for insulin injections because of medications like metformin and sulfonylureas.

Our knowledge of type 2 diabetes has continued to grow over the last several decades, thanks to research. More individualized and successful treatment plans have been made possible by the discovery of genetic markers linked to the illness, the understanding of the function of inflammation and the gut microbiota, and the creation of new pharmacological classes.

The Present Context and Difficulties: It is now understood that type 2 diabetes is a complicated, multifaceted illness that has elements of both the environment and heredity. Despite significant advancements in our knowledge of the condition, type 2 diabetes remains difficult to prevent and treat, especially in low- and middle-income nations where access to healthcare and education is constrained.

Once thought to be an adult-onset disorder, type 2 diabetes is increasingly being diagnosed in children and adolescents. This underscores the critical need for public health programs that target obesity and sedentary lifestyles early in life.

Further research and international cooperation will be required to halt the Type 2 diabetes pandemic and improve the prognosis of people afflicted with the illness.

1.3 Type 2 Diabetes's Global Impact

Type 2 diabetes is now one of the biggest threats to public health in the twenty-first century. Its effects are felt not only by people but also by economies, communities, and healthcare systems around the globe.

Incidence and Prevalence
Over the last several decades, there has been a significant increase in the incidence of type 2 diabetes. The International Diabetes Federation (IDF) projects that 643 million individuals (20–79 years old) will have diabetes globally by 2021, up from an anticipated 537 million in 2021.

Diabetes prevalence is on the rise, particularly in low- and middle-income countries, where obesity and diabetes rates are on the rise due to sedentary lifestyles, rapid urbanization, and dietary changes. In many of these nations, higher rates of complications and death result from the healthcare systems' inadequacy, which makes them ill-equipped to manage the rising load of chronic illnesses.

Impact on the Economy: The financial toll that type 2 diabetes takes is enormous. According to IDF predictions, the amount spent on diabetes treatment globally in 2021 will reach \$966 billion, a 316% rise over the previous 15 years. This amount accounts for both direct costs—such as hospital stays, prescription drugs, and medical care—and indirect costs—such as missed work, absenteeism, and early retirement owing to disability.

The expense of controlling diabetes places a heavy strain on healthcare systems in high-income nations. For instance, one in every four healthcare dollars in the US is spent on treating diabetes, making it the most costly chronic illness. The whole economic burden is increased by the expense of controlling diabetic consequences such as renal disease, cardiovascular disease, and amputations.

The effects on the economy are significantly more pronounced in low- and middle-income nations. Diabetes patients sometimes have to pay large out-of-pocket costs for their prescription drugs and medical care, which may be financially difficult and limit their access to essential therapies. Poverty and economic inequality are made worse when someone loses their job due to an illness or an early death.

Impact on Society and Culture: Additionally, type 2 diabetes has significant social and cultural consequences.

Food plays a major role in social and familial interactions in many cultures; therefore, implementing the dietary adjustments needed to treat diabetes may be difficult. The way diabetes is seen and treated may also be influenced by cultural customs and beliefs. For instance, there could be a stigma attached to diabetes in certain cultures, which prevents people from getting treatment or from telling others they have the illness.

There are now more difficulties since Type 2 diabetes in kids and teenagers is on the increase. In addition to dealing with the difficulties of growing up, young individuals with diabetes have to deal with the added burden of maintaining a chronic illness. Concern about the long-term effects of early-onset diabetes on mental and physical health is rising.

International Proposals and Reactions: Numerous programs have been initiated by governments, non-governmental organizations, and international organizations to tackle the worldwide diabetes pandemic. Diabetes has been given top priority by the World Health Organization (WHO) in its global action plan for the prevention and management of non-communicable diseases (NCDs).

The Sustainable Development Goals (SDGs) were approved by the UN in 2016, and one of the goals is to cut the premature death rate from NCDs—including diabetes—by one-third by 2030. To achieve this goal, it will take coordinated efforts to address socioeconomic determinants of health, encourage healthy behaviors, and increase access to healthcare.

Numerous nations have started public health campaigns with the goals of increasing knowledge about diabetes risk factors, encouraging frequent screenings, and supporting a balanced diet and physical exercise. In order to delay the development of type 2 diabetes and lessen the severity of its effects, these initiatives are crucial.

Technology and Innovation's Role: Technological developments have also been essential in controlling Type 2 diabetes's worldwide effects. People may now better control their diabetes thanks to the invention of insulin pumps, mobile health applications, and continuous glucose monitoring devices.

Access to diabetes treatment has increased because of telemedicine and digital health platforms, especially in rural or underdeveloped regions. With the use of these technologies, medical professionals can now give patients individualized advice, assistance with lifestyle modifications, and real-time condition monitoring.

For those with type 2 diabetes, research into novel therapies, including SGLT2 inhibitors and GLP-1 receptor agonists, has produced more efficient management choices. These drugs not only lower blood sugar levels but also lower the risk of kidney and cardiovascular problems.

Although type 2 diabetes has an unavoidable worldwide effect, there is still hope for the future. More research, technological advancements, and public health campaigns are opening doors for improved care, prevention, and eventually a cure for this widespread illness.

There is hope that raising awareness and stepping up efforts to fight Type 2 diabetes may help reverse the present trends and lower the disease's worldwide burden. To do this, people, governments, healthcare organizations, and communities everywhere must work together.

UNDERSTANDING THE SCIENCE BEHIND TYPE 2 DIABETES

2.1 The Role of Insulin in the Body

Insulin is often referred to as the "key" that unlocks the doors of our cells to allow glucose, the body's primary source of energy, to enter. This vital hormone is produced by the pancreas, an organ nestled behind the stomach, and it plays a crucial role in maintaining the delicate balance of blood sugar levels.

How Insulin Works

After you eat a meal, your digestive system breaks down carbohydrates into glucose, which is then absorbed into the bloodstream. As blood glucose levels rise, the pancreas responds by releasing insulin. This insulin binds to receptors on the cell surface, signaling them to open up and allow glucose to enter. Once inside the cells, glucose can be used immediately for energy or stored for future use, primarily in the liver and muscles, in the form of glycogen.

Insulin also plays a role in fat metabolism. It encourages fat cells (adipocytes) to take in glucose and convert it into fat for storage. Additionally, insulin inhibits the breakdown of fat in adipose tissue, ensuring that the body uses available glucose as its primary energy source rather than tapping into fat stores.

In a healthy individual, this system works seamlessly, maintaining blood glucose levels within a narrow range, typically between 70 and 140 mg/dL. After the cells absorb glucose, blood sugar levels drop, prompting the pancreas to reduce insulin secretion. This feedback loop ensures that blood glucose levels remain stable, preventing the highs and lows that can lead to health complications.

The importance of insulin sensitivity

For this system to function correctly, the body's cells must be sensitive to insulin. Insulin sensitivity refers to how effectively cells respond to the presence of insulin. When cells are highly sensitive to insulin, they require only a small amount of the hormone to absorb glucose from the blood. Conversely, when cells become less responsive to insulin—a condition known as insulin resistance—more insulin is needed to achieve the same effect.

High insulin sensitivity is beneficial, as it helps maintain stable blood sugar levels with minimal insulin production. However, when insulin sensitivity decreases, the pancreas must work harder to produce more insulin to keep blood sugar levels in check. Over time, this increased demand can exhaust the pancreas, leading to a decline in insulin production and the eventual onset of type 2 diabetes.

The Role of Insulin Beyond Blood Sugar Control

While insulin's primary function is to regulate blood sugar, it also influences other physiological processes. For example, insulin affects protein synthesis in muscles, promoting muscle growth and repair. It also plays a role in how the body stores and uses fat, influencing body weight and composition.

Insulin's influence extends to the brain as well, where it affects appetite and food intake. Research suggests that insulin signaling in the brain helps regulate hunger and satiety, contributing to the overall balance of energy intake and expenditure.

Given insulin's wide-ranging effects on the body, any disruption in its production or action can have significant consequences, as seen in the development and progression of type 2 diabetes.

2.2 Insulin Resistance: Causes and Effects

Insulin resistance is a key feature of type 2 diabetes and one of the earliest signs that something is amiss in the body's metabolism. When the body's cells become resistant to insulin's effects, it sets off a cascade of events that ultimately leads to the development of diabetes. Understanding the causes and effects of insulin resistance is crucial for grasping the underlying science of type 2 diabetes.

What is insulin resistance?

Insulin resistance occurs when the cells in the body's muscles, fat, and liver start to ignore or "resist" the signal from insulin to take up glucose from the blood. As a result, glucose remains in the bloodstream, leading to elevated blood sugar levels. To compensate, the pancreas produces more insulin, trying to overcome the resistance and maintain normal blood sugar levels.

Initially, this extra insulin production, known as hyperinsulinemia, may keep blood sugar levels within a normal range. However, as insulin resistance worsens, the pancreas may struggle to produce enough insulin, leading to higher blood sugar levels and, eventually, the diagnosis of type 2 diabetes.

Causes of Insulin Resistance

Several factors contribute to the development of insulin resistance, many of which are interconnected:

Genetics: A family history of type 2 diabetes increases the likelihood of developing insulin resistance. Certain genetic variations can affect how the body responds to insulin, making some individuals more prone to insulin resistance than others.

Obesity: Excess body fat, particularly around the abdomen, is a significant risk factor for insulin resistance. Fat cells, especially visceral fat (fat stored around the organs), release inflammatory substances called adipokines that can interfere with insulin signaling. Additionally, excess fat can cause changes in lipid metabolism, leading to the accumulation of fat within the liver and muscles, which further impairs insulin sensitivity.

Physical Inactivity: Regular physical activity helps improve insulin sensitivity by enhancing glucose uptake in muscles and reducing the amount of fat stored in the body. Conversely, a sedentary lifestyle can lead to weight gain and an increase in insulin resistance.

Diet: A diet high in refined sugars, processed foods, and unhealthy fats contributes to insulin resistance. Excessive consumption of sugary foods and beverages leads to frequent spikes in blood sugar and insulin levels, which, over time, can cause cells to become less responsive to insulin. A diet lacking in fiber, whole grains, and healthy fats can also negatively impact insulin sensitivity.

Age: Insulin resistance tends to increase with age, possibly due to changes in body composition, hormone levels, and physical activity as people get older.

Hormonal Imbalances: Certain hormonal conditions, such as polycystic ovary syndrome (PCOS) and Cushing's syndrome, are associated with insulin resistance. These conditions can alter insulin signaling and glucose metabolism, increasing the risk of type 2 diabetes.

Chronic Stress: Prolonged stress triggers the release of stress hormones like cortisol, which can promote insulin resistance by increasing blood sugar levels and altering fat metabolism.

Effects of Insulin Resistance

The effects of insulin resistance extend beyond the risk of developing type 2 diabetes. Chronic insulin resistance can lead to a range of metabolic disturbances, often referred to as metabolic syndromes. Metabolic syndrome is a cluster of conditions that increase the risk of heart disease, stroke, and other health problems. These conditions include:

High blood pressure: Insulin resistance is associated with increased blood pressure, a major risk factor for cardiovascular disease. Insulin can affect the balance of sodium and fluid in the kidneys, leading to higher blood pressure.

Dyslipidemia: Insulin resistance can lead to abnormal levels of lipids (fats) in the blood, including elevated levels of triglycerides and low-density lipoprotein (LDL) cholesterol, as well as reduced levels of high-density lipoprotein (HDL) cholesterol. These lipid imbalances contribute to the development of atherosclerosis, a condition where plaque builds up in the arteries, increasing the risk of heart attack and stroke.

Fatty Liver Disease: Insulin resistance is strongly linked to non-alcoholic fatty liver disease (NAFLD), a condition characterized by the accumulation of fat in the liver. NAFLD can progress to more severe liver conditions, such as non-alcoholic steatohepatitis (NASH) and cirrhosis.

Increased Inflammation: Insulin resistance is associated with a state of chronic, low-grade inflammation. This inflammation can contribute to the development of various chronic diseases, including cardiovascular disease, certain cancers, and neurodegenerative disorders.

Weight Gain and Obesity: Insulin resistance can lead to weight gain, particularly in the abdominal area. This type of fat distribution, known as central obesity, is a significant risk factor for type 2 diabetes and cardiovascular disease.

Impaired Glucose Tolerance: Insulin resistance can cause impaired glucose tolerance (IGT), a condition where blood sugar levels are higher than normal but not yet high enough to be classified as diabetes. IGT is a precursor to type 2 diabetes and is often detected through an oral glucose tolerance test.

Addressing insulin resistance through lifestyle changes, such as losing weight, increasing physical activity, and improving diet, is crucial in preventing or delaying the onset of type 2 diabetes and its associated complications.

2.3 The Pancreas and Beta Cells

The pancreas is a vital organ in the regulation of blood sugar levels and plays a central role in the development of type 2 diabetes. Understanding the structure and function of the pancreas, particularly the beta cells that produce insulin, is key to understanding how type 2 diabetes develops.

Anatomy and Function of the Pancreas

The pancreas is a glandular organ located in the abdomen, behind the stomach. It has both exocrine and endocrine functions, meaning it produces enzymes for digestion (exocrine) and hormones for blood sugar regulation (endocrine).

The exocrine portion of the pancreas produces digestive enzymes that are released into the small intestine to help break down fats, proteins, and carbohydrates. These enzymes are essential for the proper digestion and absorption of nutrients.

The endocrine portion of the pancreas contains clusters of cells known as the islets of Langerhans. Within these islets, there are several types of cells, including:

Alpha Cells: These cells produce glucagon, a hormone that raises blood sugar levels by stimulating the liver to release stored glucose.

Beta Cells: Beta cells are responsible for producing and secreting insulin, the hormone that lowers blood sugar levels by facilitating glucose uptake by cells.

Delta Cells: These cells produce somatostatin, a hormone that regulates the release of both insulin and glucagon, as well as other digestive hormones.

The beta cells are of particular interest in the context of type 2 diabetes, as their function is critical to maintaining normal blood sugar levels.

The Role of Beta Cells in Insulin Production

Beta cells are highly specialized cells that constantly monitor blood sugar levels and adjust insulin production accordingly. When blood sugar levels rise, such as after a meal, beta cells respond by increasing insulin secretion. The insulin then travels through the bloodstream to signal cells in the muscles, liver, and fat to absorb glucose.

The process of insulin secretion is tightly regulated and involves several steps:

1. Glucose Sensing: Beta cells have glucose transporters on their surface that allow glucose to enter the cell. Once inside, glucose is metabolized to produce energy, leading to an increase in the cellular concentration of adenosine triphosphate (ATP), the cell's energy currency.

2. Membrane Depolarization: The increase in ATP causes potassium channels in the beta cell membrane to close, leading to membrane depolarization. This depolarization causes calcium channels to open.

3. Calcium Influx: The influx of calcium into the beta cell stimulates the release of insulin-containing granules from within the cell.

4. Insulin Secretion: Insulin is released into the bloodstream, where it travels to target tissues to promote glucose uptake.

This intricate process allows beta cells to respond rapidly and precisely to changes in blood sugar levels, ensuring that glucose is available for energy while preventing excessive increases in blood sugar.

Beta Cell Dysfunction in Type 2 Diabetes

In individuals with type 2 diabetes, beta cells often become dysfunctional, leading to inadequate insulin production and secretion. Several factors contribute to beta cell dysfunction:

Genetic Factors: Certain genetic variations can impair beta cell function and increase the risk of type 2 diabetes. These genetic factors may affect the beta cells' ability to sense glucose, produce insulin, or release insulin in response to rising blood sugar levels.

Chronic High Blood Sugar (Glucotoxicity): Prolonged exposure to high blood sugar levels can damage beta cells, reducing their ability to produce and secrete insulin. This phenomenon, known as glucotoxicity, creates a vicious cycle in which worsening blood sugar control further impairs beta cell function.

Lipotoxicity: Excess fat, particularly in the form of free fatty acids, can accumulate in beta cells and interfere with their function. This condition, known as lipotoxicity, is often seen in individuals with obesity and contributes to the development of insulin resistance and beta-cell dysfunction.

Oxidative Stress: High levels of oxidative stress, caused by an imbalance between the production of harmful free radicals and the body's ability to neutralize them, can damage beta cells and impair insulin production.

Inflammation: Chronic low-grade inflammation, often associated with obesity and insulin resistance, can lead to beta cell dysfunction. Inflammatory molecules can interfere with insulin signaling and contribute to the progressive loss of beta cell function in type 2 diabetes.

As beta cells become less effective at producing and secreting insulin, blood sugar levels begin to rise, leading to the development of type 2 diabetes. Over time, the continued loss of beta cell function can result in the need for exogenous insulin therapy to maintain blood sugar control.

The Potential for Beta Cell Regeneration

Research into beta cell regeneration and preservation is an area of active investigation, as preserving or restoring beta cell function could offer a potential cure for type 2 diabetes. Scientists are exploring various approaches, including:

Stem Cell Therapy: Researchers are investigating the potential of stem cells to regenerate beta cells. By coaxing stem cells to differentiate into insulin-producing beta cells, it may be possible to restore insulin production in individuals with type 2 diabetes.

Gene Therapy: Gene therapy approaches aim to correct the genetic defects that contribute to beta cell dysfunction, potentially restoring normal insulin production.

Immunotherapy: Some researchers are exploring the use of immunotherapy to protect beta cells from immune system attack and inflammation, thereby preserving their function.

Pharmacological Agents: Several drugs are being developed to enhance beta cell function, improve insulin secretion, and protect beta cells from damage.

While these approaches are still in the experimental stages, they offer hope for the future of diabetes treatment, with the potential to reverse or halt the progression of type 2 diabetes.

2.4 How Type 2 Diabetes Develops

Type 2 diabetes is a complex and multifactorial disease that develops gradually over time. The process involves a combination of genetic predisposition, environmental factors, and lifestyle choices, all of which contribute to the progressive loss of insulin sensitivity and beta cell function.

The Progression from Insulin Resistance to Diabetes

The development of type 2 diabetes typically follows a predictable course, beginning with insulin resistance and eventually leading to full-blown diabetes.

1. Insulin Resistance: The first step in the development of type 2 diabetes is the onset of insulin resistance. As discussed earlier, insulin resistance occurs when the body's cells become less responsive to insulin, leading to higher levels of insulin in the blood as the pancreas tries to compensate.

2. Compensatory Hyperinsulinemia: In the early stages of insulin resistance, the pancreas is usually able to produce enough extra insulin to maintain normal blood sugar levels. This state of compensatory hyperinsulinemia can persist for years, during which time individuals may have normal or slightly elevated blood sugar levels.

3. Impaired Glucose Tolerance: As insulin resistance worsens and beta-cell function begins to decline, the pancreas may no longer be able to keep up with the body's insulin needs. This results in impaired glucose tolerance (IGT), a condition where blood sugar levels are higher than normal but not yet high enough to be classified as diabetes.

4. Early Diabetes: As beta cell function continues to deteriorate, blood sugar levels begin to rise more significantly, leading to the diagnosis of type 2 diabetes. At this stage, individuals may experience symptoms such as increased thirst, frequent urination, fatigue, and blurred vision.

5. Progressive Beta Cell Dysfunction: Over time, the continued loss of beta cell function leads to worsening blood sugar control, requiring more intensive treatment to manage the disease. In some cases, individuals may eventually require insulin therapy to maintain blood sugar levels within a healthy range.

Risk Factors for Developing Type 2 Diabetes

Several risk factors increase the likelihood of developing type 2 diabetes. Some of these factors are modifiable, meaning they can be changed through lifestyle interventions, while others are non-modifiable.

Age: The risk of type 2 diabetes increases with age, particularly after the age of 45. However, the disease is becoming more common in younger populations due to rising rates of obesity and sedentary lifestyles.

Family History: A family history of type 2 diabetes increases the risk of developing the disease, suggesting a genetic component to its development.

Ethnicity: Certain ethnic groups, including African Americans, Hispanics, Native Americans, and Asian Americans, are at and unhealthyhigher risk of developing Type 2 diabetes.

Obesity: Excess body weight, particularly central obesity (fat around the abdomen), is a major risk factor for insulin resistance and type 2 diabetes.

Sedentary Lifestyle: Physical inactivity contributes to weight gain and insulin resistance, increasing the risk of type 2 diabetes.

Poor Diet: A diet high in processed foods, sugary beverages, fats can contribute to insulin resistance and the development of type 2 diabetes.

History of Gestational Diabetes: Women who develop gestational diabetes during pregnancy are at increased risk of developing Type 2 diabetes later in life.

Polycystic Ovary Syndrome (PCOS): Women with PCOS are at higher risk of developing insulin resistance and type 2 diabetes.

Hypertension: High blood pressure is often associated with insulin resistance and increases the risk of developing type 2 diabetes.

Dyslipidemia: Abnormal levels of cholesterol and triglycerides are associated with an increased risk of insulin resistance and type 2 diabetes.

The Role of Inflammation in Type 2 Diabetes

Chronic low-grade inflammation is increasingly recognized as a key player in the development of type 2 diabetes. Inflammation can interfere with insulin signaling and contribute to the dysfunction of beta cells, leading to insulin resistance and impaired insulin secretion.

Obesity, particularly central obesity, is a major source of chronic inflammation. Fat cells release pro-inflammatory molecules called cytokines, which can promote insulin resistance and damage beta cells. Additionally, the accumulation of fat in the liver and muscles can trigger an inflammatory response, further exacerbating insulin resistance.

The Impact of Lifestyle on Type 2 Diabetes Development

While genetics and non-modifiable risk factors play a role in the development of type 2 diabetes, lifestyle choices have a significant impact on whether or not the disease develops. Modifiable risk factors, such as diet, physical activity, and body weight, offer opportunities for prevention and intervention.

Diet: Adopting a diet rich in whole foods, such as fruits, vegetables, whole grains, and lean proteins, can help improve insulin sensitivity and reduce the risk of type 2 diabetes. Limiting the intake of processed foods, sugary beverages, and unhealthy fats is also crucial for preventing insulin resistance.

Physical Activity: Regular physical activity, such as walking, cycling, or strength training, helps improve insulin sensitivity and maintain a healthy weight. Exercise also has a positive effect on blood pressure, cholesterol levels, and overall cardiovascular health.

Weight Management: Maintaining a healthy weight, particularly by reducing excess fat around the abdomen, is one of the most effective ways to prevent insulin resistance and type 2 diabetes. Even modest weight loss can have a significant impact on insulin sensitivity and blood sugar control.

Stress Management: Chronic stress can contribute to insulin resistance and the development of type 2 diabetes. Practices such as mindfulness, meditation, and regular physical activity can help reduce stress and its impact on blood sugar levels.

This knowledge is essential for both prevention and effective management of the disease, empowering individuals to make informed choices that can improve their health and quality of life.

TYPE 2 DIABETES CAUSES AND RISK FACTORS

The multifactorial nature of type 2 diabetes is caused by a confluence of environmental, behavioral, and genetic variables. Understanding these risk factors and causes is critical for managing and avoiding the illness.

3.1 Hereditary Propensity

Genetics' Part in Type 2 Diabetes

Since type 2 diabetes often runs in families, there may be a significant hereditary component to the illness. Numerous genetic variants that raise the incidence of type 2 diabetes have been found by researchers. Different elements of metabolism, insulin production, and insulin sensitivity may be impacted by these differences.

Variations in the genes that control insulin synthesis and glucose metabolism are important hereditary variables in type 2 diabetes. For instance, there is compelling evidence linking mutations in the TCF7L2 gene to a higher risk of type 2 diabetes. This gene is essential for both the body's efficient usage of glucose and the release of insulin.

Diabetic Forms That Are Monogenic

There are rare examples of monogenic diabetes, but the majority of Type 2 diabetes cases are caused by a combination of environmental and hereditary variables. A single gene mutation causes monogenic diabetes, which usually manifests similarly to type 2 diabetes but commonly strikes at a younger age and may not be linked to obesity.

Neonatal diabetes and maturity-onset diabetes of the young (MODY) are the two most prevalent types of monogenic diabetes. Frequently mistaken for Type 1 or Type 2 diabetes, these disorders need distinct approaches to care.

Pathology and Hazard: An individual's chance of having Type 2 diabetes is greatly increased if they have a first-degree relative who has the illness. If both of the parents have type 2 diabetes, the risk is much greater. This family risk is likely caused by a mix of common environmental variables, such as nutrition and lifestyle, as well as shared genetic characteristics.

Type 2 Diabetes and Epigenetics: In addition to conventional hereditary variables, epigenetics plays a significant role in the development of type 2 diabetes. Changes in gene expression that do not include modifications to the underlying DNA sequence are referred to as epigenetic changes. These alterations may be influenced by environmental variables such as stress, physical activity, and food.

For instance, exposure to inadequate nutrition during pregnancy or the early years of life may result in epigenetic modifications that raise the chance of developing type 2 diabetes in later life. In a similar vein, long-term stress or exposure to pollutants in the environment may cause epigenetic changes that impact glucose metabolism and insulin sensitivity.

Repercussions for Management and Prevention: Knowing a person's genetic susceptibility to type 2 diabetes may help identify those who are more likely to develop the disease and inform individualized preventative plans. For instance, more extensive lifestyle treatments, such as consistent exercise and dietary changes, may be beneficial for those with a high family history of Type 2 diabetes in order to lower their chance of contracting the illness.

Genetic testing is an increasingly useful technique for determining who has a high hereditary risk of type 2 diabetes. Although this type of testing is not currently standard practice, it may become so as our knowledge of the genetic causes of type 2 diabetes advances.

3.2 Lifestyle Elements: Nutrition, Activity, and Obesity

Dietary Influence on Type 2 Diabetes Risk

Diet is one of the most important lifestyle variables that influence the risk of type 2 diabetes. Diets high in processed foods, sugar-filled drinks, and unhealthy fats are linked to obesity and insulin resistance, two of the main risk factors for type 2 diabetes.

The Function of Processed Foods and Sugary Drinks: Sugar-filled drinks, such as soda and fruit juices with added sugar, are especially dangerous since they quickly raise blood sugar levels. Over time, insulin resistance may result from these recurrent surges. Processed foods increase the risk of developing insulin resistance and contribute to weight gain because they are often high in harmful fats and processed carbohydrates.

Healthy Food Selections: On the other hand, type 2 diabetes may be avoided by eating a diet high in whole foods, including fruits, vegetables, whole grains, and lean meats. Because these meals have a lower glycemic index, blood sugar levels rise more slowly and gradually after eating them.

They frequently include significant levels of fiber, which may improve insulin sensitivity and aid in weight control.

Physical Activity's Role in Avoiding Type 2 Diabetes

Engaging in regular physical exercise is another important way to lower your risk of type 2 diabetes. Exercise increases insulin sensitivity, which facilitates better glucose uptake by the body's cells. Additionally, it lowers stress, helps with weight control, and enhances cardiovascular health in general.

Types of Physical Activity: It is possible to avoid Type 2 diabetes by engaging in strength training activities like bodyweight exercises or weightlifting, as well as aerobic activities like walking, jogging, or cycling. For best effects, a mix of the two forms of exercise is often advised.

The Effect of Obesity on the Risk of Type 2 Diabetes: One of the biggest risk factors for type 2 diabetes is obesity. Type 2 diabetes and insulin resistance are strongly associated with excess body fat, especially around the belly. The body's metabolism may alter as a result of obesity, making it more challenging to properly control blood sugar levels.

Isleticism and Visceral Body Fat: Fat accumulated around internal organs, or visceral fat, is more metabolically active than subcutaneous fat, which is kept under the skin and may be especially hazardous. Insulin resistance may be caused by visceral fat's production of inflammatory chemicals, which can disrupt insulin signaling.

The Impact of Losing Weight on Diabetes Risk

Even a small amount of weight reduction may have a major impact on lowering the risk of type 2 diabetes. Even a little weight loss of 5–10% of body weight will reduce blood sugar and increase insulin sensitivity. In the prevention and treatment of type 2 diabetes, losing weight should be the main objective for overweight or obese people.

Combining Exercise and Diet

Combining a balanced diet with regular exercise is the most efficient strategy to reach and stay at a healthy weight. The prevention of type 2 diabetes is more likely to be effective when lifestyle modifications focus on long-term, sustainable practices.

3.3 Age and Ethnicity's Contribution

Growing older raises the risk of type 2 diabetes, especially after age 45. A portion of this rise may be attributed to the aging-related natural decrease in insulin sensitivity. In addition, weight gain, decreased physical activity, and other risk factors that lead to the development of type 2 diabetes are more common in older people.

Why Does Age Cause a Decline in Insulin Sensitivity?: The aging process causes a decrease in insulin sensitivity due to a number of variables, such as altered body composition, decreased muscle mass, and elevated visceral fat. The function of the pancreatic beta cells, which are in charge of manufacturing insulin, is also linked to aging.

Differences in Type 2 Diabetes Risk by Ethnicity: A number of ethnic groups, including Asian Americans, Native Americans, African Americans, and Hispanics, are more likely to acquire type 2 diabetes. A complex interplay of genetic, environmental, and social variables accounts for these discrepancies.

Hereditary Propensities Among Ethnic Groups: A substantial portion of the greater incidence of type 2 diabetes in certain ethnic groups may be attributed to genetic susceptibility. People of South Asian heritage, for instance, are more likely to be genetically predisposed to central obesity and insulin resistance, both of which raise the risk of type 2 diabetes.

Ambient and Socioeconomic Factors: Certain ethnic groups have a greater incidence of type 2 diabetes due to socioeconomic and environmental variables. In some neighborhoods, there is a greater prevalence of obesity, poor physical activity, and restricted access to healthy food options, all of which raise the risk of type 2 diabetes.

Cultural Affects on Lifestyle and Nutrition: Dietary and lifestyle decisions that impact the risk of type 2 diabetes are also influenced by cultural variables. Lower levels of physical exercise, combined with traditional diets high in processed carbs and fats, may raise the risk of illness.

Tackling Ethnic Differences in Diabetes Prevention: The particular difficulties that various ethnic groups confront must be considered in Type 2 diabetes prevention efforts. Reducing the incidence of Type 2 diabetes in these communities requires culturally sensitive therapies that target particular food practices, levels of physical activity, and socioeconomic constraints.

3.4 Social and Environmental Factors Affecting Health

Our living conditions have a significant impact on many aspects of our health, including our risk of developing type 2 diabetes. The term "environmental factors" refers to a broad category of variables, including exposure to toxins and pollution levels, as well as the availability of nutritious food and chances for physical exercise. These variables often interact with social determinants of health, including socioeconomic position, educational attainment, and access to healthcare, to form a complex network of factors that impact a person's risk of type 2 diabetes.

Access to Healthy Options and the Food Environment: The food environment is one of the most important environmental variables impacting the development of type 2 diabetes. In many localities, especially in low-income areas, there is limited availability of reasonably priced, healthy food. Known as "food deserts," these regions don't have any supermarkets or grocery shops that provide fresh produce, whole grains, and fruits. Alternatively, locals could depend on fast food restaurants or convenience shops, which mostly sell processed meals that are heavy in fat, sugar, and refined carbs. The chance of bad eating habits, weight gain, and ultimately insulin resistance and Type 2 diabetes is increased by this restricted access to nutrient-dense foods.

On the other hand, populations with a lower incidence of Type 2 diabetes tend to have easier access to healthier dietary alternatives, such as fresh produce at grocery stores and farmers' markets. Community gardens, mobile markets, and nutrition education programs are a few examples of initiatives that provide access to healthy foods and may significantly lower the incidence of type 2 diabetes in underprivileged communities.

Environment for Physical Activities: The physical environment also has a significant influence on the risk of type 2 diabetes through affecting levels of physical activity. Regular physical activity might be discouraged in neighborhoods lacking parks, walking trails, and recreational facilities—safe and convenient places to exercise. For example, citizens may be less inclined to walk or bike for fitness or transportation if the town has few sidewalks or is seen as hazardous owing to high crime rates. This sedentary way of life raises the risk of type 2 diabetes, obesity, and insulin resistance.

Walking communities, bike lanes, and public parks are key components of urban design that may encourage physical activity and lower the prevalence of type 2 diabetes. Programs that provide free or inexpensive access to sports facilities, gyms, and fitness courses may also support people in low-income neighborhoods in maintaining an active lifestyle and a healthy weight.

Toxin Exposure and Pollution: According to recent studies, exposure to certain chemicals and environmental pollutants may also contribute to the development of type 2 diabetes. For instance, there is evidence connecting air pollution to a higher risk of type 2 diabetes and insulin resistance. A common air pollutant called fine particulate matter (PM2.5) may cause inflammation in the body, which can hinder insulin signaling and result in insulin resistance.

Similarly, there is a link between a higher risk of obesity and Type 2 diabetes and exposure to endocrine-disrupting chemicals (EDCs), which include phthalates, bisphenol A (BPA), and several pesticides. These substances have the potential to disrupt hormone balance and metabolism, which may result in insulin resistance and weight gain.

Coordinated actions at the local, national, and international levels are necessary to reduce exposure to environmental contaminants and poisons. Public health can be safeguarded, and the prevalence of type 2 diabetes may be decreased with the support of policies that control air quality, prohibit the use of dangerous chemicals, and advance clean energy.

Health Determinants in Society: Type 2 diabetes risk is significantly influenced by social determinants of health, such as social support, education, employment, and socioeconomic position. Disparities in health outcomes across various demographic groups are typically caused by the intersection of these variables with environmental factors.

Demographic Position and Diabetes Risk: Type 2 diabetes is more likely to strike those with lower socioeconomic status (SES). Numerous variables, such as restricted access to healthcare, a diet high in nutrients, and possibilities for physical exercise, contribute to this elevated risk. Chronic stress is also more common in those with lower socioeconomic status (SES) because of issues with housing, employment, and financial instability. Long-term stress may result in unhealthy coping strategies, including binge eating, smoking, or abusing alcohol, all of which raise the risk of type 2 diabetes.

Furthermore, a person's capacity to get and comprehend health information may be impacted by their lower SES, which is often linked to lower levels of education. Controlling diabetes risk factors, such as food and exercise, and seeking prompt medical attention may be more difficult if there is a lack of health literacy.

Training and Profession: Education level is another important factor that influences the risk of type 2 diabetes. Greater levels of education are often linked to improved health outcomes, such as a decreased risk of type 2 diabetes. In addition to influencing health-related habits like food and exercise, education may provide people with the information and abilities they need to successfully navigate the healthcare system. Higher-educated people are also more likely to work in positions that provide paid time off for illness, health insurance, and other advantages that promote wellness.

Occupation is another factor that influences diabetes risk. Occupations that are physically taxing or require extended periods of inactivity might raise the risk of type 2 diabetes and obesity. For instance, those who have professions that demand a lot of sitting, such as truck drivers or office workers, may be more vulnerable because of their physical inactivity. However, physically taxing occupations involving heavy lifting or repeated movements might result in long-term discomfort or injuries that restrict one's ability to exercise and increase body weight.

Mental Health and Social Support: A key component of controlling and preventing type 2 diabetes is social support. Strong social networks, which include friends, family, and neighborhood associations, increase an individual's likelihood of adopting healthy habits and seeking medical attention when necessary. In addition to offering practical and emotional support, social support may help manage the day-to-day problems of living with Type 2 diabetes, including taking medicines, maintaining an active lifestyle, and following a nutritious diet.

Diabetes risk and socioeconomic determinants of health are intimately related to mental health. People with a poor socioeconomic position and little social support are more likely to suffer from depression, anxiety, and chronic stress. It may be more challenging to maintain good habits and successfully manage diabetes as a result of certain mental health issues. Improving outcomes for those at risk of or already suffering from Type 2 diabetes requires integrated methods that address diabetes treatment and mental health.

3.5 Type 2 Diabetes and Gestational Diabetes: A Connection

Understanding Diabetes During Pregnancy

Pregnancy-related diabetes usually goes away once the baby is delivered and is known as gestational diabetes. It is, nonetheless, a significant risk factor for the later onset of type 2 diabetes. When a woman's body cannot create enough insulin to meet the increased demands of pregnancy, she develops gestational diabetes, which is characterized by raised blood sugar levels. Routine glucose screening tests are used to identify this issue, which often manifests in the second or third trimester of pregnancy.

Gestational Diabetes Risk Factors: Being overweight or obese, having a family history of diabetes, and belonging to certain ethnic groups like African Americans, Hispanics, Native Americans, or Asian Americans are some of the variables that raise the chance of developing gestational diabetes. Women who have given birth to a big baby (more than 9 pounds) or who have had gestational diabetes during a prior pregnancy are also more vulnerable.

The Relationship Between Type 2 Diabetes and Gestational Diabetes: Type 2 diabetes is far more likely to strike women who have gestational diabetes in the future. Up to 50% of women with gestational diabetes, according to research, may go on to acquire Type 2 diabetes five to ten years after delivering a child. Although the precise processes causing this elevated risk are not entirely known, a mix of genetic, hormonal, and lifestyle variables are thought to be involved.

Insulin Resistance and Dysfunction of Beta Cells: Because gestational diabetes is a sign of insulin resistance and beta cell malfunction, it often precedes the onset of type 2 diabetes. The effects of placental hormones during pregnancy raise the body's need for insulin, which may make it more challenging for the body to control blood sugar levels. Pregnant women are more likely to have underlying insulin resistance or beta cell malfunction, which may worsen into gestational diabetes.

Type 2 diabetes may develop as a result of insulin resistance, which does not go away after pregnancy, and a continued decrease in beta cell activity. Because excess body fat and insulin resistance are strongly related, women who were overweight or obese before becoming pregnant are more at risk.

The Significance of Postpartum Care: Women who have had gestational diabetes must undergo routine follow-up treatment after pregnancy due to the substantial correlation between gestational diabetes and type 2 diabetes. In addition to counseling on lifestyle modifications to lower the risk of diabetes, this care should include blood sugar monitoring to watch for the onset of type 2 diabetes. Key tactics for avoiding Type 2 diabetes following gestational diabetes include consuming a balanced diet, remaining physically active, and maintaining a healthy weight.

Affect on the Youngster: Offspring of moms diagnosed with gestational diabetes are also more likely to have obesity and Type 2 diabetes in their later years. While the intrauterine environment may also have an impact, genetic factors account for a portion of this risk. Elevated blood sugar levels in pregnancy may cause the baby to develop too quickly and accumulate more fat, which might put the infant at risk for metabolic problems.

In children born to moms with gestational diabetes, early therapies such as breastfeeding promotion, good eating habits encouragement, and physical activity assistance may help lower the incidence of obesity and type 2 diabetes.

It is crucial to comprehend Type 2 diabetes's causes and risk factors for both therapy and prevention. The condition is mostly determined by genetic predisposition, lifestyle choices, including nutrition and exercise, and environmental and social determinants of health. Furthermore, gestational diabetes is an important risk factor that may provide early indicators of type 2 diabetes in the future. Through focused treatments and lifestyle modifications, people may improve their general health and well-being and lower their chance of acquiring type 2 diabetes.

IDENTIFYING TYPE 2 DIABETES SYMPTOMS

4.1 Typical type 2 diabetes symptoms

Since many patients with type 2 diabetes may not exhibit symptoms until the condition has advanced noticeably, the illness is sometimes referred to as "silent killer." But there are a number of typical symptoms that might indicate Type 2 diabetes, and it's important to identify these early indicators so that treatment can begin as soon as possible.

Frequent urination (polyuria) is one of the most prevalent symptoms. When blood sugar levels are high, the kidneys work overtime to filter and absorb more sugar. Increased urination results from the extra sugar being expelled into the urine by the kidneys when they are unable to handle it, bringing fluids from the tissues with it. This may interfere with sleep, especially at night.

Increased thirst (polydipsia) is another symptom strongly associated with frequent urination. Thirst is a signal to stimulate fluid intake when the body loses more fluids via urine. Undiagnosed Type 2 diabetes patients may find this cycle of frequent urination and thirst to be very draining.

Another sign is ***explained weight loss***; however, this is more often linked to Type 1 diabetes. Nonetheless, weight loss is a possible side effect for certain Type 2 diabetics, particularly if the disease is causing insufficient insulin production or impaired insulin use. This causes fat and muscle to be broken down for energy, which causes weight reduction.

Fatigue is a prevalent symptom that has several causes, but in the case of type 2 diabetes, it often results from the body's inefficient utilization of glucose as an energy source. People experience a sharp decline in energy when their cells are deprived of glucose, which makes them feel drained and listless.

Blurred vision may occur when blood sugar levels are too high, causing the eye's lens to expand and impair focus for a short time. If left untreated, this could result in more severe consequences, such as diabetic retinopathy, the primary cause of blindness.

Other signs include frequent infections or slow-healing sores. Elevated blood sugar levels may impede blood flow and impact the body's inherent recuperative mechanism. This may raise the risk of infection and result in chronic sores, especially on the feet. Furthermore, elevated blood sugar creates the perfect habitat for yeast and bacteria, which increases the likelihood of infections, particularly in the urinary system, skin, and gums.

Neuropathy, or tingling or numbness in the hands and feet, is another symptom that often remains undiagnosed until it becomes worse. High blood sugar may cause nerve damage over time, which can cause tingling, burning, or numbness in the affected limbs. In addition to discomfort, this nerve injury might result in muscular weakness.

Acanthosis nigricans, or "darkened skin patches, often develop in the groin, armpits, or neck folds. These deep, velvety skin patches are often a symptom of insulin resistance and a prelude to the onset of type 2 diabetes.

Another typical symptom is hunger, which is also sometimes called polyphagia. Because their bodies can't properly utilize the food they consume for energy, people with type 2 diabetes may still feel hungry even after eating more. This may worsen the disease by triggering a vicious cycle of overeating and weight gain.

4.2 Early diagnosis is critical

It is impossible to exaggerate the significance of an early Type 2 diabetes diagnosis. When Type 2 diabetes is discovered later in life, the body's systems and organs may have already suffered grave harm. Prolonged high blood sugar may cause major side effects such as heart disease, kidney damage (nephropathy), nerve damage (neuropathy), and eye damage (retinopathy). These issues may possibly be fatal and have a major negative influence on quality of life.

Early detection prevents complications

Timely action, which may either postpone or avoid the start of problems, is made possible by early diagnosis. Through early diagnosis and treatment of type 2 diabetes, people may take charge of their health and lower their chance of long-term consequences. Early intervention often consists of blood sugar-controlling drugs in addition to lifestyle modifications such as eating a better diet, getting more exercise, and decreasing weight.

Improving Results with Prompt Intervention

Research has shown that treating type 2 diabetes at an early age may enhance results and lower the likelihood of complications. For instance, the United Kingdom Prospective Diabetes Study (UKPDS) showed that strict blood sugar management dramatically lowered the incidence of microvascular complications, such as kidney and eye impairment, among individuals with recently diagnosed Type 2 diabetes. In addition to improving long-term blood sugar management, early therapy may help sustain the function of the pancreatic cells known as beta cells, which are responsible for producing insulin.

The Function of Medical Professionals in Early Diagnosis

Early detection of type 2 diabetes is greatly aided by

healthcare practitioners. Regular screening helps find the condition before symptoms worsen, particularly for those who are at high risk. People who are overweight or obese, have a family history of diabetes, are over 45, or are members of certain ethnic groups—such as African Americans, Hispanics, Native Americans, or Asian Americans—should get screening in particular.

4.3   Diagnostic Procedures and Tests

FPG Test: Fasting Plasma Glucose: One of the most commonly used tests for the diagnosis of type 2 diabetes is the fasting plasma glucose (FPG) test. After at least eight hours of fasting, the blood sugar level is measured using this test. Less than 100 mg/dL is the usual blood sugar level when fasting. Pre-diabetes is defined as a level of 100 to 125 mg/dL, and type 2 diabetes is confirmed by two different tests with a result of 126 mg/dL or above.

The OGTT (Oral Glucose Tolerance Test): Another diagnostic test for type 2 diabetes is the Oral Glucose Tolerance Test (OGTT), which is especially useful when the findings of the FPG test are unclear. Blood sugar levels are measured using the OGTT both before and two hours after ingesting a drink high in glucose. Less than 140 mg/dL is regarded as normal blood sugar, but pre-diabetes is indicated by a number between 140 and 199 mg/dL. Type 2 diabetes is confirmed by a result of 200 mg/dL or above.

A1C Test: The glycated hemoglobin test, or A1C test, gives an average of the blood sugar levels over the previous two to three months. This test calculates the proportion of hemoglobin—the oxygen-carrying protein in red blood cells—that is coated with sugar, or glycated. A1C levels between 5.7% and 6.4% suggest pre-diabetes; 5.7% to 6.4% is deemed normal; and 6.5% or above on two different tests confirms a Type 2 diabetes diagnosis.

Positive Glucose Random Test: Without requiring a fast, blood sugar levels may be measured at any time of day with the random plasma glucose test. When diabetic signs like increased thirst, frequent urination, and unexplained weight loss are present, this test is often done. Type 2 diabetes may be confirmed by a blood sugar level of 200 mg/dL or greater, in addition to the symptoms of the disease.

Pre-Diabetes Screening and Early Intervention: Pre-diabetic screening is crucial for Type 2 diabetes prevention and early intervention. Pre-diabetics have higher blood sugar levels than usual, but they are not high enough to be considered diabetic. Early identification of pre-diabetes enables lifestyle modifications that may stop or slow the onset of type 2 diabetes. These adjustments include eating a healthier diet, getting more exercise, and decreasing weight.

4.4 Pre-Diabetes: Alert Signals and Avoidance

What Is Diabetes Precursor?

Blood sugar levels that are higher than usual but not high enough to be classified as type 2 diabetes are known as pre-diabetes. Because it offers a window of opportunity for prevention, pre-diabetes is a critical stage in the development of type 2 diabetes. At this point, the body starts to exhibit symptoms of insulin resistance, a condition in which cells lose their sensitivity to insulin, raising blood sugar levels.

Danger Indices of Potential Diabetes

Pre-diabetes is hard to identify without a blood test. Pre-diabetes may be present, however, as indicated by a few warning signals. These include having a sedentary lifestyle, being over 45, having a family history of Type 2 diabetes, and being overweight or obese, especially with extra fat around the belly. Furthermore, pre-diabetes is more common in several ethnic groups, including Asian Americans, Native Americans, African Americans, and Hispanics.

Additional possible indicators of insulin resistance include darker skin patches (acanthosis nigricans) in the groin, armpits, and neck. Pre-diabetes is also more likely to develop in women who have had gestational diabetes during pregnancy or who gave birth to a child weighing more than nine pounds.

Modifying Your Lifestyle to Avoid Type 2 Diabetes

The good news is that lifestyle modifications may typically prevent or postpone the onset of type 2 diabetes and treat pre-type 2 diabetes. A mere 5% to 7% reduction in body weight may have a substantial impact on lowering the incidence of type 2 diabetes. Frequent exercise, like walking, swimming, or cycling for five days a week for at least half an hour, may also help decrease blood sugar levels and increase insulin sensitivity.

blood sugar levels.

Preventing type 2 diabetes may also be greatly aided by eating a balanced diet low in processed foods, sugar-filled beverages, and red meats and high in whole grains, fruits, vegetables, lean proteins, and healthy fats. Reducing alcohol use and giving up smoking may also help to minimize the risk.

The Function of Drugs in the Management of Pre-Diabetes
Healthcare professionals may sometimes suggest medication to treat pre-diabetes and stop it from developing into type 2 diabetes. The most often given drug for pre-diabetes is metformin, since it increases insulin sensitivity and lowers blood sugar levels. Nonetheless, lifestyle modifications continue to be the mainstay of managing pre-diabetes, and medication is usually used in addition to these adjustments.

Observation and Frequent Examinations
Pre-diabetics should see their doctor on a regular basis to evaluate their blood sugar levels and determine their risk of acquiring type 2 diabetes. Frequent monitoring allows for

timely modifications to lifestyle choices and, if necessary, drug regimens to prevent the condition from getting worse.

STRATEGIES FOR DAY-TO-DAY MANAGEMENT

5.1 Establishing a Harmonious Schedule

Maintaining a healthy balance in many areas of daily life, such as nutrition, exercise, medication, and stress reduction, is necessary for people with type 2 diabetes. Developing a regular routine that aids in maintaining stable blood sugar levels is one of the most crucial tactics. This entails eating meals on a regular basis, exercising, taking prescribed drugs, and keeping an eye on blood sugar levels.

Nutritious Eating Practices

In order to effectively manage type 2 diabetes, a diet is essential. A nutritious diet that includes whole grains, fruits, vegetables, lean meats, and healthy fats will help control blood sugar levels. Portion management is critical, especially with regard to carbs, since they have the most effect on blood sugar. Low-glycemic foods, such as legumes, whole grains, and non-starchy vegetables, are especially advantageous since they release glucose gradually and reduce blood sugar rises.

Planning meals is another important tactic. When hunger hits, the temptation to reach for less healthy alternatives may be avoided by planning meals in advance and selecting nutritious snacks. Making educated dietary decisions may also be aided by reading food labels and knowing the amount of carbohydrates in various meals.

Daily Exercise

Exercise is another crucial component of managing type 2 diabetes. Because exercise increases insulin sensitivity and improves the muscles' ability to use glucose, blood sugar levels are lowered. Regular exercise, such as cycling, swimming, walking, or resistance training, may help you manage your diabetes and enhance your general health.

It's critical to select long-term, sustainable activities that you enjoy. Make gradual changes to your fitness routine by starting with small, manageable goals, such as going for a quick walk after meals. Finding small ways to fit exercise into your daily life—like using the stairs instead of the elevator—can have a significant impact over time. Consistency is the key.

Reduction of Stress

Blood sugar levels can be significantly impacted by stress. Stress causes the body to release adrenaline and cortisol, two hormones that can increase blood sugar. As a result, stress management is a crucial component of daily diabetes care. Deep breathing, yoga, meditation, and mindfulness are a few methods that can help lower stress and enhance general wellbeing.

Furthermore, it's critical to obtain adequate sleep, since insufficient sleep may raise stress levels and disturb blood sugar levels. Create a calming bedtime routine and stick to a regular sleep schedule to achieve your daily goal of 7-9 hours of quality sleep.

Building a Support System

Living with Type 2 diabetes can be challenging, but having a strong support system can make a significant difference. Family, friends, and healthcare professionals can provide emotional support, practical advice, and encouragement. Joining a diabetes support group, either in person or online, can also be beneficial, as it offers the opportunity to connect with others who are facing similar challenges.

5.2 Monitoring Blood Sugar Levels

Why Monitoring Matters

Regularly monitoring blood sugar levels is a cornerstone of controlling type 2 diabetes. It gives essential information on how diet, exercise, medicine, and stress impact your blood sugar levels. By monitoring these levels, you can make educated judgments about your day-to-day management and take action to avoid issues.

Self-Monitoring Tools

The most common technique for self-monitoring is using a blood glucose meter, a tiny instrument that measures the amount of glucose in a drop of blood, which is usually collected via a finger prick. Continuous Glucose Monitors (CGMs) are also available, which offer real-time blood sugar measurements throughout the day and night. CGMs are very helpful in seeing patterns and trends in blood sugar levels, which enables more accurate control.

It's crucial to heed the advice of your medical professional regarding how frequently to check your blood sugar. While some people might need to check their levels several times a day, others might only need to do so infrequently. You and your healthcare provider can spot patterns and make the necessary adjustments if you and your log include notes about your diet, exercise routine, and medications.

Blood Sugar Target Ranges

Your healthcare provider will give you target blood sugar ranges based on your individual needs. Typically, the desired range before meals is between 80 and 130 mg/dL, and less than 180 mg/dL two hours after meals. However, these objectives may vary based on variables such as age, general health, and the existence of other medical disorders.

It's vital to strive for these goal ranges as regularly as possible, since maintaining blood sugar levels within these ranges may help avoid consequences such as heart disease, kidney damage, nerve damage, and eye difficulties.

Interpreting Results and Making Adjustments

Interpreting blood sugar readings involves understanding how various factors affect your levels. For example, if your blood sugar is higher than usual after a meal, it may indicate that you consumed more carbohydrates than your body can handle. On the other hand, low blood sugar levels might suggest that you need to adjust your medication or eat more frequently.

It's important to address any persistent trends of high or low blood sugar with your healthcare provider. They can help you adjust your diet, exercise regimen, or medication dosage as part of your treatment plan.

A1C Testing's Role

In addition to daily monitoring, the A1C test offers an overall view of your blood sugar management over the preceding two to three months. This test calculates the proportion of hemoglobin—the oxygen-carrying protein in red blood cells—that is coated with sugar, or glycated. For most people with type 2 diabetes, an A1C level below 7% is ideal, but depending on your unique situation, your healthcare provider may have a different objective in mind.

5.3 Insulin and Medication's Role

Oral Pharmaceuticals

For many people with type 2 diabetes, oral medications play a crucial role in managing blood sugar levels. There are several types of oral medications available, each working in different ways to help control blood sugar. Common classes of diabetic medicines include:

Metformin: Often the first medication prescribed, metformin works by reducing glucose production in the liver and improving insulin sensitivity.

Aspartame: The pancreas produces more insulin in response to these medications. Examples are glipizide and glyburide.

DPP-4 inhibitors: By supporting the body's innate ability to lower blood sugar, these medications mainly lower blood sugar by increasing the release of insulin after meals. Examples include sitagliptin and saxagliptin.

SGLT2 inhibitors: These medications assist the kidneys in excreting excess glucose from the blood into the urine. Examples include canagliflozin and dapagliflozin.

Thiazolidinediones: These medications increase the body's sensitivity to insulin. Pioglitazone and rosiglitazone are two examples.

Based on your individual requirements, your healthcare professional will choose the best prescription, considering your lifestyle, blood sugar levels, and any other medical issues you may have.

Insulin Therapy

While Type 2 diabetes is often managed with oral medications and lifestyle changes, some individuals may require insulin therapy to achieve optimal blood sugar control. Insulin is a hormone that helps the body use glucose for energy, and in Type 2 diabetes, the body may not produce enough insulin or may be resistant to its effects.

There are several types of insulin, categorized by how quickly they start to work and how long their effects last. These include:

Rapid-acting insulin: Begins to work within 15 minutes and lasts for about 3 to 5 hours. It is typically taken before meals.
Short-acting insulin: It takes around 30 minutes to start functioning and lasts for 5 to 8 hours. It is also taken before meals.
Intermediate-acting insulin: It takes 1 to 2 hours to start working and lasts for 12 to 18 hours. It is often used in combination with short- or rapid-acting insulin.
Long-acting insulin provides a steady level of insulin for up to 24 hours and is typically taken once or twice a day.

Insulin can be administered using a syringe, an insulin pen, or an insulin pump. How much, when, and how to use insulin will be advised by your doctor. It's important to follow their instructions closely to avoid complications such as hypoglycemia (low blood sugar).

Combination Therapy

In some cases, a combination of oral medications and insulin may be necessary to achieve optimal blood sugar control. Combination therapy can be tailored to your specific needs, and your healthcare provider will work with you to develop the most effective treatment plan.

Managing medication side effects

Like all medications, diabetes medications can have side effects. Common side effects include gastrointestinal issues such as nausea, diarrhea, and stomach pain, especially with metformin. Sulfonylureas can cause low blood sugar (hypoglycemia), while SGLT2 inhibitors may increase the risk of urinary tract infections.

If you experience any side effects, it is critical to notify your healthcare provider so that they can modify your treatment plan to reduce the severity of these effects. Never stop taking your medication without consulting your healthcare provider, as this could lead to uncontrolled blood sugar levels and increase the risk of complications.

5.4 Understanding Hypoglycemia and Hyperglycemia

Hypoglycemia (low blood sugar)

Hypoglycemia occurs when blood sugar levels drop below normal, often below 70 mg/dL. This can happen if you take too much insulin, skip a meal, or engage in intense physical activity without adjusting your food intake or medication. Symptoms of hypoglycemia may include:

Trembling or shaking; sweating
Lightheadedness or dizziness; confusion or trouble focusing; hunger; irritability; weakness or exhaustion; blurred eyesight

While severe, hypoglycemia may result in convulsions, unconsciousness, or possibly a coma. It's critical to identify hypoglycemia symptoms early and take prompt measures to elevate blood sugar levels. This may be done by taking fast-acting carbs, such as glucose tablets, fruit juice, or ordinary soda.

If you experience frequent episodes of hypoglycemia, it's important to discuss this with your healthcare provider. They can help adjust your treatment plan to reduce the risk of low blood sugar.

Hyperglycemia (High Blood Sugar)

Hyperglycemia occurs when blood sugar levels are too high, typically above 180 mg/dL. This can happen if you eat too much, don't take enough insulin or medication, are ill, or are under stress. Symptoms of hyperglycemia may include:

Increased thirst, frequent urination, exhaustion, headache, blurred vision, and difficulty focusing

Untreated hyperglycemia may result in life-threatening complications, including diabetic ketoacidosis (DKA), which is characterized by the body burning down fat for energy and producing an accumulation of acids in the blood called ketones.

Monitoring your blood sugar levels often, taking your medicine as directed, and adhering to your food plan are all important aspects of managing hyperglycemia. It's critical to let your healthcare practitioner know if your blood sugar levels are consistently high, because they may need to modify your treatment strategy.

5.5 Psychological Effects of Living with Diabetes

Emotional Challenges: Living with type 2 diabetes may take a toll on your mental well-being. The ongoing need to check blood sugar levels, control food, and take medicine may be stressful. Anxiety, despair, and irritation are common emotions among diabetics. It's very unusual to experience a feeling of loss or sadness about the lifestyle modifications necessary to treat the disease.

It's important to recognize these emotions and ask for help when you need it. Speaking with a counselor or therapist who focuses on chronic disease may help you strengthen your emotional resilience and create coping mechanisms. In addition to offering a feeling of belonging and comprehension, support groups facilitate connections with like-minded individuals.

Diabetes Exhaustion: The emotional weariness that may result from the ongoing challenges of controlling diabetes is known as "diabetes burnout." Burnout may manifest as not taking care of one's blood sugar, not taking one's medicine as prescribed, or not following one's diet. It's critical to get assistance if you're feeling burned out. Together, you and your healthcare practitioner may identify strategies to lessen the stress of managing your diabetes and enhance your general quality of life.

The Significance of Introspection: It's essential to engage in self-compassion practices if you have type 2 diabetes. It's easy to get angry or to put the responsibility on oneself for changes in blood sugar levels or for any "failures" in controlling the illness. But it's crucial to keep in mind that managing diabetes is a difficult and continuous process, and the achievement of perfection is not the aim.

Your mental health may be greatly improved by treating yourself with kindness, having reasonable expectations, and acknowledging and appreciating your tiny successes. Keep in mind that you don't have to go through this trip alone, and it's OK to seek assistance.

Developing an Upbeat Attitude: You may approach diabetes treatment with a feeling of empowerment rather than defeat by cultivating a positive mentality. You may feel more in control of your health by concentrating on the areas you can manage, such as your food, exercise routine, and prescription drugs. Creating attainable objectives, like lowering your A1C or increasing the amount of physical exercise in your daily routine, may also keep you motivated.

It's critical to understand that maintaining type 2 diabetes is a journey rather than a sprint. There will be ups and downs along the road, but you can overcome the difficulties and have a happy, fulfilled life with diabetes if you adopt a positive outlook and ask for help when you need it.

THE VALUE OF A WELL-BALANCED DIET

6.1 Diabetic Management Foundation

Effective management of type 2 diabetes is based on a balanced diet. Making educated food choices is crucial because what you eat has a direct impact on your blood sugar levels. In addition to helping to stabilize blood sugar levels, maintain a healthy weight, and avert complications related to diabetes, a balanced diet gives your body the nutrients it needs to function at its best.

A varied diet that provides vital nutrients like vitamins, minerals, fiber, protein, and healthy fats is part of a balanced diet for people with type 2 diabetes. This variety ensures that your body gets what it needs while also making eating more enjoyable, which makes it easier to stick to your diet over the long run.

Parts of a well-balanced diet
The following food groups are included in a well-rounded diet:

Leafy greens, broccoli, cauliflower, peppers, tomatoes, and other non-starchy vegetables should make up half of your plate. These have a low calorie and carb content but a high fiber, vitamin, and mineral content that helps control blood sugar and keep you feeling full.
Fruits: Although they naturally contain sugars, fruits also offer important nutrients like antioxidants, fiber, and vitamins. Choose whole fruits over processed ones, such as pears, apples, and berries, as they have a lower glycemic index and are less likely to spike blood sugar. As moderation is essential, pay attention to portion sizes.

To help control blood sugar levels, opt for whole grains rather than refined grains. High-fiber whole grains, such as brown rice, quinoa, oats, and whole wheat bread, slow down the digestion and absorption of carbohydrates, thereby averting abrupt spikes in blood sugar levels.

Lean proteins, such as turkey, chicken, fish, tofu, beans, and lentils, may help you feel fuller for longer periods of time and keep your blood sugar levels steady. Protein is essential for building and repairing tissues and has little effect on blood sugar.

Healthy Fats: A variety of foods, including avocados, nuts, seeds, olive oil, and fatty seafood like salmon, are good sources of fats. These fats have the potential to lower inflammation, promote heart health, and provide long-lasting energy without raising blood sugar levels.

Dairy products, including yogurt, milk, and cheese, may be included in a balanced diet as long as they are low in fat or have no fat. Select fortified dairy substitutes like soy yogurt or almond milk if you're lactose-intolerant or would rather eat a plant-based diet.

Portion Control: An essential part of controlling Type 2 diabetes is portion management. Consuming significant amounts of even healthful meals might cause blood sugar rises. Effective portion control can be achieved by using instruments such as food scales, measuring cups, or visual aids such as comparing portion sizes to typical objects.

Just follow the "plate method" to make sure your meals are well-balanced. Place non-starchy vegetables on half of your plate, lean protein on the other quarter, and whole grains or starchy vegetables on the remaining quarter. You can have a balanced meal that helps you control your blood sugar by adding a serving of fruit or dairy on the side.

6.2 Using the Glycemic Index to Count Carbs

Knowing Your Carbohydrates: Though they are the body's main energy source, carbohydrates also have the most effect on blood sugar levels. Your body converts carbohydrates into glucose when you eat them, which enters the bloodstream and raises blood sugar levels. For those who have type 2 diabetes, this means that controlling their carbohydrate intake is essential.

Bread, pasta, rice, cereals, fruits, vegetables, dairy products, and sweets are just a few of the foods that contain carbohydrates. Sugars, starches, and fibers are the three primary categories into which they fall. Fiber lowers blood sugar levels, whereas sugars and starches do. In fact, fiber can aid in blood sugar stabilization by delaying glucose absorption.

Carbohydrate Quantification: One useful technique for controlling blood sugar levels is carb counting. You keep a record of the grams of carbs you eat at each meal and snack. This technique assists you in maintaining a steady carbohydrate intake throughout the day and helps you anticipate how your blood sugar will react to various foods.

To begin counting carbohydrates, do the following:

1. Learn which foods contain carbohydrates and how much of them you should eat each day by reading "Learn the Basics. A small apple has roughly 20 grams of carbohydrates, compared to the typical 15 grams found in one slice of bread.

2. **Set Your Carbohydrate Goals:** Based on your unique requirements, degree of activity, and treatment plan, collaborate with your physician or a certified dietitian to establish your daily carbohydrate target. Your meals and

snacks will each count toward this objective.

3. **Check nutrition labels:** Nutrition labels provide important information regarding the amount of carbohydrates in packaged goods. Observe the "Total Carbohydrate" column, which comprises fiber, sugars, and starches. The "net carbs," or the carbohydrates that have an impact on blood sugar, are obtained by deducting the fiber content from the total amount of carbohydrates.

4. **Use Apps and Tools:** With numerous apps and web resources, you can keep track of your carbohydrate intake with the aid of numerous apps and web resources. These programs frequently include databases of foods and their carbohydrate contents, which makes it simpler to keep track of your meals and adhere to your carbohydrate targets.

Grade-Level Index: A carbohydrate-containing food's rate of blood sugar rise is compared to pure glucose, which has a GI of 100, using a ranking system called the glycemic index (GI). Blood sugar rises more slowly and gradually in response to foods with a low GI (55 or below) than in response to meals with a high GI (70 or above).

Including low-GI foods in your diet will assist you in better controlling your blood sugar levels. Examples of low-GI foods are as follows:

Whole grains such as oats, quinoa, and barley
Chickpeas, black beans, and lentils are examples of legumes.
Broccoli, cauliflower, and other non-starchy vegetables

All fruits, such as berries, pears, and apples

Combining Foods to Improve Blood Sugar Regulation

Blood sugar response can be regulated by combining foods with different GI values, such as high-GI foods and low-GI foods, or carbohydrates, protein, and fat. For slow down the absorption of carbohydrates and avoid blood sugar spikes, for instance, include a source of protein, such as chicken or beans, in a meal that includes rice.

6.3: Organizing Your Meals to Maintain Blood Sugar Levels

The Value of Regular Meal Timing
Eating at regular intervals throughout the day helps maintain stable blood sugar levels. Skipping meals or eating large meals infrequently can lead to blood sugar fluctuations, which can be challenging to manage. Ideally, you should strive to eat three balanced meals a day, with healthy snacks in between if required.

Consistent meal timing helps regulate insulin levels and ensures that your body has a steady supply of glucose for energy. If you take insulin or other diabetes medications, eating meals at the same time each day can help prevent low blood sugar (hypoglycemia) or high blood sugar (hyperglycemia).

Creating a Diabetes-Friendly Meal Plan

A well-structured meal plan for Type 2 diabetes focuses on nutrient-dense foods, portion control, and balance. Here's how to construct one:

1. **Plan Ahead:** Preparing meals in advance will help you make better choices and avoid the temptation of less nutritious alternatives. Batch cooking, meal preparation, and establishing a shopping list may streamline the process and guarantee you have nutritious meals ready to go.

2. **Balance Your Plate:** As mentioned earlier, the plate method is a simple way to create balanced meals. Incorporate a variety of vegetables, lean proteins, whole grains, and healthy fats into each meal.

3. **Include Snacks Wisely:** Healthy snacks may help reduce blood sugar falls between meals. Choose snacks that contain protein, fiber, and healthy fats, such as a small handful of nuts, a piece of fruit with a dollop of nut butter, or yogurt with a sprinkle of seeds.

4. **Mind Your Portions:** Use portion control tools, such as measuring cups or visual aids, to keep your servings in check. For instance, one-half cup, or about the size of a tennis ball, is the standard portion size for cooked pasta.

5. **Remain Hydrated:** Drinking enough water is critical for maintaining good health and controlling blood sugar levels. Choose water or other calorie-free beverages over sugary drinks, and try to drink at least eight glasses of water each

day.

Flexible meal scheduling: Flexibility is just as important as structure in managing type 2 diabetes. Life is unpredictable, and there will be times when you eat out, attend social events, or face unexpected changes in your routine. The goal is to make the best choices possible in these situations and not stress about occasional deviations from your meal plan.

When dining out, search for menu choices that suit your dietary rules, such as grilled meats, steamed vegetables, and salads with dressing on the side. Don't be hesitant to request alterations to suit your preferences, such as switching fries for a side salad or asking for sauces on the side.

6.4 The Role of Fiber, Protein, and Fats

Fiber: The Blood Sugar Stabilizer
Fiber is a type of carbohydrate that the body cannot digest, meaning it does not raise blood sugar levels. Instead, fiber helps to slow sugar absorption and improve blood sugar control. There are two types of fiber: soluble and insoluble.

Soluble Fiber: Dissolves in water and forms a gel-like substance in the digestive tract. This particular kind of fiber lowers cholesterol and blood sugar. Good sources include oats, barley, legumes, apples, and citrus fruits.

Insoluble Fiber: Does not dissolve in water and adds bulk to the stool, promoting regular bowel movements. It also helps you feel full, which can aid in weight management. Sources of insoluble fiber include whole grains, nuts, seeds, and vegetables like carrots, cucumbers, and tomatoes.

Incorporating high-fiber foods into your diet can help you maintain stable blood sugar levels, improve digestion, and support heart health. Aim for at least 25–30 grams of fiber per day, and increase your intake gradually to avoid digestive discomfort.

Protein: The Satiety Enhancer
Protein plays a crucial role in diabetes management because it helps to regulate blood sugar levels and keep you feeling full between meals. Protein is a vital part of a balanced diet because, in contrast to carbohydrates, it has little effect on blood sugar levels.

Sources of lean protein include:

Poultry (chicken, turkey)
Fish (tuna, cod, and salmon)
– Eggs
Low-fat dairy (Greek yogurt, cottage cheese)
Plant-based proteins (tofu, tempeh, legumes, nuts, seeds)

Incorporating protein into each meal and snack can help stabilize blood sugar levels and reduce the likelihood of overeating. For example, pairing an apple with a handful of almonds or adding grilled chicken to a salad can help you stay satisfied and avoid blood sugar spikes.

Healthy Fats: The Heart Protectors
Healthy fats are an essential element of a diabetes-friendly diet. They provide essential fatty acids, support cell function, and help the body absorb fat-soluble vitamins (A, D, E, and K). Healthy fats can also improve insulin sensitivity and reduce inflammation, both of which are important in managing type 2 diabetes.

Sources of healthy fats include:
Monounsaturated Fats: Found in olive oil, avocados, and nuts. These fats can help lower undesirable cholesterol (LDL) and raise beneficial cholesterol (HDL).

Polyunsaturated Fats: Found in fatty fish (salmon, mackerel, and sardines), walnuts, flaxseeds, and chia seeds. These fats contain omega-3 and omega-6 fatty acids, which improve heart health and prevent inflammation.

Omega-3 Fatty Acids: Omega-3s, a specific type of polyunsaturated fat, are particularly beneficial for people with type 2 diabetes. They help reduce the risk of heart disease, which is a common complication of diabetes. Sources include fatty fish, flaxseeds, chia seeds, and walnuts.

Incorporating healthy fats into your meals can help you feel satisfied and provide long-lasting energy. For example, drizzle olive oil on your salad, add avocado to your sandwich, or snack on a handful of nuts.

6.5 Managing Sugar Cravings and Emotional Eating

Understanding sugar cravings

People with type 2 diabetes may find it very difficult to control their sugar cravings. Biological, psychological, and environmental variables often work together to fuel these urges. When you consume sugar, your brain releases dopamine, a neurotransmitter associated with pleasure and reward. This can create a cycle where you crave more sugar to achieve the same pleasurable feeling.

However, controlling sugar cravings is critical to maintaining blood sugar levels and avoiding problems. Understanding the underlying causes of these cravings can help you develop strategies to reduce them.

Strategies to Manage Sugar Cravings

1. Eat balanced meals: Ensuring that your meals contain a balance of protein, fiber, and healthy fats can help stabilize your blood sugar levels and reduce cravings. When your body is well-nourished, you're less likely to experience intense sugar cravings.

2. Stay hydrated: Sometimes, thirst is mistaken for hunger or cravings. Drinking adequate water throughout the day may help avoid dehydration and lower the chances of sugar cravings.

3. **Choose Natural Sweeteners**: If you're craving something sweet, opt for natural sweeteners like stevia or monk fruit, which do not raise blood sugar levels. You can also satisfy your sweet tooth with naturally sweet foods like fruit, which contain fiber and essential nutrients.

4. **Eat With Mindfulness:** Eating mindfully can increase your enjoyment of your food and help you feel satisfied with smaller portions. It also helps you pay attention to your hunger cues. Recognizing when you're eating for stress or boredom instead of actual hunger is another benefit of mindful eating.

5. **Keep nutritious snacks on hand:** Having nutritious, low-sugar snacks that are easily accessible may help you avoid the temptation of sugary foods. Some options include a handful of nuts, a piece of fruit with nut butter, or a small serving of Greek yogurt with berries.

6. **Get Enough Sleep:** Lack of sleep may boost desires for sugary foods as your body seeks immediate sources of energy. Aim for 7-9 hours of sleep per night to support your overall health and reduce sugar cravings.

Emotional Eating and Its Triggers
Emotional eating happens when you use food to deal with emotions rather than to fulfill hunger. Emotional eating frequently involves consuming high-sugar or high-fat foods

that can cause blood sugar spikes, so this can be especially difficult for those who have Type 2 diabetes.

Common triggers for emotional eating include stress, boredom, loneliness, and anxiety. Recognizing these triggers is the first step in breaking the cycle of emotional eating.

Strategies for Managing Emotional Eating

1. **Find Your Triggers:** Maintain a journal to monitor your feelings and eating habits. You can use this to pinpoint particular circumstances or emotions that trigger emotional eating.

2. **Try healthy alternatives:** Instead of turning to food for consolation, try alternate methods to deal with your emotions. This could entail going for a stroll, doing deep breathing techniques, giving a friend a call, or picking up a fun hobby.

3. **Empathize with Yourself:** Treat yourself nicely if you make a mistake and start eating emotionally. It's critical to understand that managing diabetes is a journey and that obstacles will inevitably arise. Focus on learning from the event and making better choices going forward.

4. **Seek Support:** If emotional eating is a recurrent difficulty, consider talking with a therapist or counselor who specializes in eating disorders or chronic diseases. They may help you address the underlying emotional problems that lead to emotional eating and create coping mechanisms.

5. **Set realistic goals:** Setting small, attainable goals will help you develop confidence and make long-lasting changes when it comes to managing your diabetes and emotional eating. Honor your accomplishments, no matter how little, and keep striving for a more positive connection with food.

Developing a Nutritious Connection with Food
A vital component of managing Type 2 diabetes is cultivating a positive relationship with food. This entails viewing food as a source of sustenance rather than guilt or tension. Finding balance, savoring your food, and making decisions that promote your general wellbeing are key.

Remember that it's good to have an occasional treat, as long as it fits within your overall meal plan and doesn't contribute to blood sugar spikes. The key is moderation and attentiveness. By having a healthy connection with food, you can take control of your diabetes and enjoy a meaningful life.

PHYSICAL ACTIVITY AND EXERCISE

Physical activity and exercise are essential parts of controlling type 2 diabetes. Regular physical exercise lowers the risk of diabetes-related problems, improves overall well-being, and helps regulate blood sugar levels. The advantages of exercise, how to design a successful fitness program, the many forms of exercise, and useful advice for maintaining an active lifestyle while managing diabetes will all be covered in this part.

7.1 Advantages of Consistent Exercise

Enhanced blood sugar regulation

Improved blood sugar management is one of the biggest advantages of regular exercise for those with type 2 diabetes. Exercise raises insulin sensitivity, so your cells can use glucose more efficiently when you exercise because it raises insulin sensitivity. Exercise helps reduce blood sugar levels because it causes your muscles to absorb glucose from the circulation without the need for insulin.

Frequent exercise may also aid in lowering insulin resistance, a problem that many Type 2 diabetics have. Exercise may help with blood sugar management by increasing insulin sensitivity and reducing the need for medication.

Control of Weight

Type 2 diabetes must be managed by maintaining a healthy weight, and weight control is greatly aided by frequent exercise. Exercise promotes weight loss or maintenance by increasing metabolism, burning calories, and building lean muscle mass.

Even a modest weight loss of 5% to 10% of body weight may have a big impact on insulin resistance, blood sugar regulation, and the likelihood of complications from diabetes.

Health of the Heart

Heart attacks and strokes are among the cardiovascular diseases that people with type 2 diabetes are more likely to experience. Frequent exercise lowers blood pressure, raises beneficial cholesterol (HDL), and lowers negative cholesterol (LDL). These effects all contribute to improved cardiovascular health.

Exercise also reduces the risk of atherosclerosis, or the accumulation of fatty deposits in the arteries; strengthens the heart; and improves circulation. Regular physical exercise may considerably lower the risk of cardiovascular problems in patients with type 2 diabetes by increasing heart health.

Emotional and Mental Health
Exercise is beneficial for mental and emotional health in addition to physical health. The body's natural mood enhancers, endorphins, are released when physical exercise is undertaken and may help lower stress, anxiety, and despair.

Treating the psychological effects of type 2 diabetes is just as crucial for patients as treating the physical symptoms. Frequent exercise may enhance happiness, increase self-worth, and give one a feeling of accomplishment—all of which are factors that lead to a higher standard of living.

Increased adaptability and mobility
Maintaining flexibility and mobility as we age is crucial, particularly for those with type 2 diabetes, who may be more susceptible to joint issues or decreased mobility. Frequent exercise increases muscular strength, balance, and joint flexibility, all of which lead to increased mobility and a decreased chance of falling.

Maintaining an active lifestyle and participating in everyday activities is facilitated by increased mobility and flexibility, both of which are essential for the long-term treatment of diabetes.

Decreased Potential for Problems
Frequent exercise may help lower the chance of developing kidney disease, retinopathy (eye damage), neuropathy (nerve damage), and other issues linked to type 2 diabetes. Exercise enhances circulation, supports overall organ function, and reduces the risk of nerve and tissue damage.

Exercise is essential for the long-term treatment of type 2 diabetes because it lowers the risk of complications and promotes a better, more meaningful life for those with the condition.

7.2 Formulating an Exercise Program for the Management of Diabetes

Making Reasonable Objectives
Setting reasonable objectives based on your current fitness level, medical history, and personal preferences is crucial before beginning an exercise program. First, decide what you want to accomplish with exercise: better blood sugar regulation, weight loss, improved cardiovascular health, or just remaining active.

Tracking your progress and maintaining motivation may be facilitated by creating SMART goals—specific, measurable, realistic, relevant, and time-bound. A SMART goal may be to exercise for thirty minutes every day for five days a week or to drop ten pounds in three months.

Talking with Your Medical Staff

It's crucial to speak with your healthcare team before starting a new fitness regimen, particularly if you have any pre-existing medical illnesses or difficulties with type 2 diabetes. Your physician may suggest certain safety measures or adjustments, as well as assist you in determining the safest and most beneficial forms of exercise for your circumstances.

For instance, your doctor may suggest avoiding high-impact workouts that might injure your legs or feet if you have neuropathy. Your doctor may advise beginning with low-intensity activities and progressively increasing the intensity as your fitness level increases if you have cardiovascular problems.

Choosing the Appropriate Exercise Forms

Aerobic activity, weight training, and flexibility exercises are just a few of the activities that should be included in a comprehensive exercise program for controlling type 2 diabetes. Combining several forms of exercise may help you reach your best health goals since they each have special advantages.

When selecting workouts, take your lifestyle and personal preferences into account. Long-term adherence to a fitness regimen is higher when the activities you participate in are enjoyable. Choose hobbies that you love and can include in your daily schedule, such as yoga, cycling, swimming, or walking.

Growing Gradually and Beginning Slowly

If you've never worked out before or haven't been active in a long time, it's crucial to begin carefully and build up to longer and more intense exercises. Start with low-impact exercises like swimming or walking, and try to limit your sessions to 10 to 15 minutes.

Gradually increase the length and intensity of your exercises as your fitness level rises. The goal is to increase weekly moderate-intensity aerobic activity to at least 150 minutes, with strength training activities occurring at least twice a week.

Keep an eye on blood sugar levels

It's critical to check your blood sugar levels before, during, and after physical activity, because exercise may alter them. This is particularly true if you're on medication or insulin. You may modify your medicine, diet, or exercise regimen as needed by understanding how your body reacts to various forms of activity.

Before going out, if your blood sugar is too low (less than 100 mg/dL), have a little snack to bring it back up to a safe level. Exercise should be avoided until your blood sugar levels drop to a safer range if they are excessively high (over 250 mg/dL), particularly if you have ketones in your urine.

7.3 Exercise Types: Strength Training, Aerobics, and Flexibility

Exerts in Aerobics

Aerobic exercise, also referred to as cardiovascular or cardio exercise, is a series of rhythmic, continuous movements that raise your heart rate and strengthen your heart. People with type 2 diabetes may benefit most from aerobic exercise since it lowers blood sugar, increases insulin sensitivity, and promotes weight reduction.

Typical aerobic workout regimens consist of:

Walking: Walking is one of the most simple and convenient aerobic exercises. It is almost always portable, doesn't need any specialized gear, and is adaptable to many degrees of fitness.

Cycling: Cycling is a low-impact workout that strengthens the legs and improves cardiovascular fitness. It may be done outside or on a stationary cycle.

Swimming: People with arthritis or joint discomfort may greatly benefit from swimming, as it is a full-body exercise that is light on the joints.

Dancing: Dancing is an enjoyable and social approach to increasing heart rate while improving flexibility and coordination.

Aim for at least 150 minutes of moderate-intensity aerobic activity per week, or 30 minutes a day, five days a week. If you've never worked out before, begin with shorter workouts and work your way up to longer ones as your fitness level rises.

Intense Conditioning

Exercises that develop and preserve muscle mass are part of strength training, sometimes referred to as resistance or weight training. Because muscle tissue is more insulin-sensitive than fat tissue, strength training is beneficial for people with type 2 diabetes because it may help reduce blood sugar levels. In addition, strength training increases bone density, aids in weight control, and improves general physical function.

Typical strength training regimens consist of:

Weightlifting: targeting various muscle groups with workouts using weight machines or free weights like barbells or dumbbells in the gym.

Bodyweight Exercises: Push-ups, squats, lunges, and planks use your own body weight as resistance.

Resistance Bands: Exercises may be performed at home or on the go by using elastic bands as resistance.

Aim to include strength training activities that target all main muscle groups at least twice or three times a week for the best results. As your strength increases, progressively increase the resistance by starting with smaller weights or resistance bands.

Adaptability and extension

Stretching and yoga are two types of flexibility exercises that can increase range of motion, reduce the risk of injury, and encourage relaxation. Flexibility exercises may help people with type 2 diabetes maintain healthier joints, feel less tight in their muscles, and move about more freely. Your routine may benefit from including flexibility exercises to help lower stress and enhance mental health.

Typical flexibility exercises consist of the following:

Static Stretching: To lengthen muscles and increase flexibility, hold stretches for 15 to 30 seconds.
Dynamic Stretching: performing a range of motion movements before an activity to warm up muscles and improve flexibility.
Yoga: Enhance flexibility, balance, and mental clarity via a mind-body practice that blends strength, stretching, and relaxation methods.

At least twice or three times a week, when your muscles are heated and more malleable after strength or cardio training, include flexibility exercises in your regimen.

7.4: Keeping Active Despite Diabetes: Useful Advice

Exercise regimens or gym visits are not necessarily necessary to maintain an active lifestyle for those with type 2 diabetes. Including physical exercise in your everyday routine may be a more flexible and manageable strategy, particularly if you have a hectic schedule or would rather be active on the go. These useful hints can assist you in incorporating exercise into your everyday routine.

1. **Profit from Everyday Opportunities**

It is possible to incorporate physical exercise into daily work so that being active doesn't require additional time. Over the course of a day, little adjustments like parking further away from entrances, walking or cycling for quick errands, and using the stairs rather than the elevator may add up to a substantial amount of exercise.

If you work at a desk, stand up and move every hour. You may increase your energy levels and break up extended periods of sitting with as little as a few minutes of stretching or walking. When it's feasible, try having meetings while standing or utilizing a standing desk.

2. Turn household chores into an exercise

Doing household tasks like gardening, cleaning, and yard maintenance may be beneficial methods to maintain an active lifestyle. Exercises that demand physical exertion and may raise your heart rate include cleaning, mopping, raking leaves, and shoveling snow.

Play some upbeat music and have some fun. You may make cleaning more intense and enjoyable by pushing yourself to do jobs faster or by dancing as you clean.

3. Utilize Technology to Remain Inspired

Several applications and gadgets can help you measure your exercise levels and maintain motivation. Apps for smartphones, pedometers, and fitness monitors may measure your heart rate, count your steps, and send you reminders to move throughout the day.

To help you reach your weekly or daily exercise objectives, set up technological support. For extra incentive and accountability, a lot of applications come with challenges, awards, and social features that let you interact with friends or join groups.

4. Divide your work into brief sessions

If you struggle to dedicate long periods of time to working out, consider dividing your workouts into shorter bursts throughout the day. For instance, instead of doing a single

30-minute exercise, try three 10-minute walks. With this strategy, it may be easier to fit in exercise while maintaining the necessary daily physical activity intake.

Your blood sugar levels and general health may benefit from even modest levels of exercise. Finding ways to exercise frequently throughout the day is more critical than the duration or intensity of each session. Consistency is the key.

5. Include Friends and Family

Involving others makes being active more pleasurable and sustainable. Ask your friends, colleagues, or family to accompany you on bike rides, walks, or exercise courses. Exercise partners may provide encouragement, accountability, and support, which can help you maintain your fitness regimen.

Engage your kids in physical activities such as playing sports, hiking, or park play if you have children. This encourages you to maintain your level of activity and provides a positive example for living a healthy lifestyle.

6. Discover interest-based activities

Finding something you enjoy is the best way to stay active. Engaging in activities you like, such as dance, swimming, hiking, or yoga, facilitates commitment. Explore different exercises until you find one that works for you.

If you are a person who likes change, consider adding some

new activities to your schedule. Cross-training, or doing several forms of exercise on different days, may help lower the chance of injury and avoid boredom.

7. Make sensible plans and acknowledge your accomplishments

Establishing attainable and reasonable objectives is essential for long-term success. Begin with modest, doable objectives, like walking more steps each day or incorporating an extra few minutes of exercise into your weekly schedule. Gradually increase the length, frequency, or intensity of your exercises as you become better.

Honoring your accomplishments, no matter how little, may keep you inspired and confident. Acknowledging your efforts, whether it's by buying new gym attire, taking a well-deserved day off, or just putting in the effort, is crucial to keeping momentum going.

8. Respond to difficulties and pay attention to your body

Because life is unpredictable, there may be periods when maintaining an active lifestyle is more difficult. Having a hectic schedule, being sick, or being hurt might make it tough to stick to your regular regimen. At these times, it's critical to be adaptable and adjust your level of activity to the circumstances at hand.

When your body tells you to, prioritize rest and recuperation. If your normal routine is out of the question, think about performing softer exercises like stretching, strolling, or quick yoga sessions. Recall that maintaining an active lifestyle is a lifetime adventure, and it's OK to modify your regimen as necessary.

9. Remember to be safe

Safety is crucial while continuing an active lifestyle with type 2 diabetes. To avoid injury, always warm up before working out and cool down afterward. If you have neuropathy, make sure to wear suitable footwear to protect your feet. Additionally, make sure to stay hydrated by drinking plenty of water before, during, and after physical exercise.

Before and after exercise, check your blood sugar levels and carry a fast-acting carbohydrate, such as fruit juice or glucose pills, in case your blood sugar falls too low. Exercise should be stopped right away if you feel lightheaded, breathless, have chest discomfort, or have any other strange symptoms. If needed, get medical help.

10. Develop an activity habit

Making physical activity a regular part of your life is the best strategy for staying active. Whether it's working out in the morning, during lunch breaks, or after work, create a regimen that works for you. The more consistent you are,.

Recall that maintaining an active lifestyle with Type 2 diabetes involves more than simply treating your illness; it also entails raising your standard of living in general.

Engaging in regular physical exercise may improve your mood, make movement easier, and lead to a longer, healthier life. You may take charge of your health and flourish with Type 2 diabetes by adding exercise to your regular routine and figuring out how to stay motivated.

Drugs and Available Therapies

Effective Type 2 diabetes management sometimes requires a mix of dietary adjustments and pharmaceutical therapies. With the appropriate treatment plan, you can avoid difficulties, maintain satisfactory blood sugar levels, and live a more pleasant life.

8.1 Oral Drugs: Kinds and Mechanisms of Action

For those with type 2 diabetes, oral medicines are often the first line of therapy, particularly when dietary and activity modifications alone are insufficient to regulate blood sugar levels. These drugs function in various ways to assist in controlling blood sugar, enhance insulin sensitivity, and lower the chance of problems.

Categories of Oral Drugs

1. The Biguanides, or Metformin: One of the most often recommended drugs for type 2 diabetes is metformin. It works by decreasing the liver's production of glucose and enhancing the body's sensitivity to insulin. This lowers blood sugar levels without significantly increasing body weight. When blood sugar management is required, metformin is often the first medicine given. It is typically taken once or twice a day with meals.

2. Sulfonylureas: Sulfonylureas are another family of oral drugs that stimulate the pancreas to produce more insulin. Glipizide, glyburide, and glimepiride are a few examples. These medications effectively reduce blood sugar levels and are usually given before meals. Careful monitoring is required because it can sometimes lead to hypoglycemia, or low blood sugar, and weight gain.

3. DPP-4 Inhibitors: Sitagliptin and saxagliptin are examples of dipeptidyl peptidase-4 (DPP-4) inhibitors. These medications function by raising the levels of incretin hormones, which aid in the body's production of more insulin when needed and decrease the quantity of glucose that the liver releases. In general, DPP-4 inhibitors are well tolerated and less likely to result in hypoglycemia.

4. SGLT2 Inhibitors: Canagliflozin and dapagliflozin are examples of sodium-glucose co-transporter 2 (SGLT2)

inhibitors that reduce blood sugar by forcing the kidneys to excrete extra glucose in the urine. These drugs not only decrease blood sugar but also cut the risk of heart disease and encourage weight reduction. On the other hand, they could make dehydration and UTIs more likely.

5. Thiazolidinediones (TZDs): Pioglitazone and rosiglitazone are examples of thiazolidinediones that increase insulin sensitivity by increasing the body's cells' sensitivity to the hormone. These medicines are often used in conjunction with other prescriptions and have the ability to reduce blood sugar levels. They are often recommended cautiously since they may result in weight gain, fluid retention, and an increased risk of heart failure.

6. Meglitinides: Meglitinides, such as nateglinide and repaglinide, act similarly to sulfonylureas in inducing an increase in pancreatic production. They help control blood sugar rises and are fast-acting; they are given before meals. Compared to sulfonylureas, they may cause fewer bouts of low blood sugar because they are shorter-acting.

7. Inhibitors of Alpha-Glucosidase: Acarbose and miglitol are examples of alpha-glucosidase inhibitors that function by slowing down the intestinal breakdown of carbs, thereby reducing the risk of severe blood sugar increases after meals. These drugs are taken as soon as you bite into a meal, and they are often given in addition to other diabetic drugs.

How Cooperative Oral Drugs Are

To get the best blood sugar management, a variety of oral drugs are often used in combination. Targeting several elements of blood sugar management, including insulin sensitivity, glucose absorption, and the generation of insulin, is made possible by this method. The optimal combination will be decided by your doctor depending on your specific requirements, overall health, and how effectively each medicine controls your blood sugar.

Please Note: Always Ask your doctor for permission and advice before taking any drugs.
In order to effectively manage Type 2 diabetes with oral drugs, continuous collaboration with your healthcare professional is essential. Every drug has a unique set of advantages, disadvantages, and possible adverse effects. To ensure your treatment is safe and effective, your doctor will consider your medical history, other health issues, and medications.

Consult your doctor before beginning, stopping, or altering your prescription regimen. They will advise you on the proper dose, when to take it, and any safety measures that should be followed while taking these drugs. In order to manage any potential adverse effects or interactions and make any changes to the treatment plan, regular follow-ups and monitoring are critical.

8.2 Insulin Therapy: Optimal Timing and Approach

Oral drugs alone may not be enough for certain Type 2 diabetics to maintain ideal blood sugar levels. In these circumstances, insulin treatment may be required. By enabling glucose to enter the body's cells and be utilized as fuel, the hormone insulin helps control blood sugar levels.

Is insulin therapy necessary?

Insulin treatment is usually taken into account when:

- Despite changing one's lifestyle and using oral drugs, blood sugar levels stay high.
- Certain laboratory tests reveal evidence of a severe insulin deficit.
- The pancreas can no longer generate enough insulin by itself.
- Tight blood sugar management is required because of a pregnancy or other health issue.

Depending on a patient's demands, insulin treatment may be started at any stage of type 2 diabetes. It may be used as a long-term remedy when other therapies are no longer effective or as a temporary measure when blood sugar levels are difficult to manage, such as during sickness or stressful situations.

Insulin Types

Different insulin types are categorized according to their rate of onset, time of peak, and duration of action. Among the primary kinds are:

1. Insulin with rapid action: Insulin lispro, aspart, and glulisine are examples of rapid-acting insulin that starts to act within 15 minutes of injection, peaks in 1-2 hours, and lasts for 3-5 hours. In order to prevent blood sugar spikes, it is usually taken prior to meals.

2. Insulin that Acts Quickly: Regular insulin, sometimes referred to as short-acting insulin, begins to function in 30 minutes, peaks in 2-4 hours, and lasts for 6–8 hours. It is typically taken half an hour before eating.

3. Insulin with Intermediate Action: Insulin that is intermediate-acting, like NPH insulin, begins to function in 1-2 hours, peaks in 4–12 hours, and lasts for 12–18 hours. To provide baseline insulin coverage, it is typically taken once or twice daily.

4. Insulin that Acts Long: Insulin glargine and insulin detemir are examples of long-acting insulins that release insulin steadily over the course of 24 hours without a noticeable peak. It is usually taken once a day to keep blood sugar levels stable

throughout the day and night.

5. Insulin Already Mixed: Pre-mixed insulin provides baseline and mealtime insulin coverage by combining two forms of insulin, often an intermediate-acting insulin and a rapid-acting insulin. It is usually taken twice a day before breakfast and supper.

How Insulin is Used

The most popular way to deliver insulin is via injection, using an insulin pump, pen, or syringe. The injection site can vary, but it is usually given in the fatty tissue of the abdomen, thigh, or upper arm. Proper injection technique is important to ensure that the insulin is absorbed correctly and to avoid discomfort or complications.

Your healthcare provider will teach you how to administer insulin, including how to measure the correct dose, where to inject, and how to store insulin. They will also help you develop a schedule that aligns with your meals, activity level, and blood sugar patterns.

Managing blood sugar with insulin

Regular monitoring of blood sugar levels is required to effectively use insulin. This helps determine how well the insulin is working and allows for adjustments to be made as needed. Your doctor may also recommend adjustments to your diet, exercise, and other medications to optimize blood sugar control.

It's important to be aware of the potential risks associated with insulin therapy, such as low blood sugar (hypoglycemia). Symptoms of hypoglycemia include dizziness, perspiration, shakiness, and disorientation. If you have these symptoms, you should ingest a fast-acting carbohydrate, such as glucose tablets or juice, and check your blood sugar levels.

8.3: New and Emerging Treatments

The area of diabetes therapy is continually expanding, with new drugs, technology, and procedures being created to improve blood sugar management and increase the quality of life for patients with type 2 diabetes.

New Pharmaceuticals

1. Opponents of GLP-1 Receptors: A more recent family of drugs called glucagon-like peptide-1 (GLP-1) receptor agonists includes dulaglutide and semaglutide, which replicate the actions of the incretin hormone GLP-1. These drugs aid in the synthesis of more insulin and decrease the release of glucagon, a hormone that elevates blood sugar) and reduce digestion, which aids in blood sugar regulation after meals. GLP-1 receptor agonists have also been shown to lower the risk of cardiovascular events and encourage weight reduction.

2. Beneficials for the Heart from SGLT2 Inhibitors: Even though SGLT2 inhibitors have been around for a while, new studies have shown that they also offer further advantages for

heart health. In addition to lowering blood sugar, medications such as canagliflozin and empagliflozin also reduce the risk of heart failure and other cardiovascular events in people with type 2 diabetes.

3. GLP-1 and GIP Dual Receptor Opponents: Currently in development is a novel family of drugs called dual glucose-dependent insulinotropic polypeptide (GIP) and GLP-1 receptor agonists. By acting on the GIP and GLP-1 receptors, these drugs increase insulin production and provide better blood sugar regulation. Preliminary research indicates that these drugs could have further advantages for cardiovascular health and weight reduction.

4. Semaglutide taken orally: GLP-1 receptor agonists have hitherto only been offered as injectable drugs. For those who would rather not utilize injections, oral semaglutide has recently been developed, offering a more practical choice. Comparable advantages are provided by oral semaglutide in terms of weight reduction, cardiovascular protection, and blood sugar regulation.

Complementary Medicines

Combination treatments aim to improve blood sugar management by combining two or more drugs with complementary mechanisms of action. Because this method addresses many facets of blood sugar management, it may be more effective than using a single medicine.

1. Combinations of Fixed Doses: Fixed-dose combos are gaining popularity; examples include metformin coupled with an SGLT2 or DPP-4 inhibitor. By lowering the total number of tablets required for therapy, these combination pills increase convenience and adherence.

2. Triple Combination Treatment: A triple combination treatment, which consists of three separate drugs with different mechanisms of action, may be advised in certain circumstances. To achieve ideal blood sugar regulation, a patient could be administered a mix of metformin, an SGLT2 inhibitor, and a GLP-1 receptor agonist.

Cutting-Edge Technologies
1. Regular Blood Sugar Monitoring (CGM): The real-time data on blood sugar levels provided by continuous glucose monitoring (CGM) devices has transformed the treatment of diabetes. These gadgets are made up of a tiny sensor that is inserted under the skin to monitor the interstitial fluid's glucose levels day and night. The information is sent to a smartphone app or receiver, enabling ongoing observation and better decision-making.

By seeing patterns and trends in blood sugar levels, CGM devices may help users avoid dangerous highs or lows by warning them before they happen. Insulin users especially benefit from this technology, as it makes dosage more accurate and improves overall control.

2. Insulin Delivery Systems Automated: Artificial pancreas systems, or automated insulin delivery systems, use a combination of an insulin pump and a continuous glucose monitor (CGM) to automatically modify insulin dosage in

response to current blood glucose levels. By decreasing the need for manual insulin changes and assisting with the maintenance of more stable blood sugar levels, these systems may lessen the stress associated with managing diabetes.

3. Intelligent Insulin Pens: Smart insulin pens, which are better than regular insulin pens, can monitor insulin dosages, provide reminders, and reveal trends in blood sugar levels by connecting to smartphone applications. These tools may reduce the risk of missing or giving the wrong dose of insulin and increase adherence.

8.4: Handling Drug Interactions and Side Effects

Despite being essential for the management of type 2 diabetes, medicines may have adverse effects or mix with other medications, causing problems. It is essential to know how to handle these problems if you want to make sure your treatment plan is secure and efficient.

Typical Adverse Reactions to Diabetes Drugs

1. Digestive Problems: One of the most often given drugs for diabetes, metformin, may have gastrointestinal side effects that include nausea, diarrhea, and cramping in the stomach. These side effects are usually minor and may go away as your body gets used to the medicine. Metformin, taken with food, might lessen these problems.

2. Low blood sugar, or hypoglycemia: Hypoglycemia, or low blood sugar, may sometimes be brought on by medications like meglitinides and sulfonylureas that boost the production of insulin. Hypoglycemia manifests as trembling, perspiration, lightheadedness, and disorientation. Eating regular meals and snacks and constantly monitoring your blood sugar levels are key to preventing hypoglycemia. If necessary, having a supply of fast-acting carbs on hand, such as juice or glucose pills, may help you swiftly boost your blood sugar.

3. Gained weight: Weight gain is a possible side effect of certain diabetic treatments, including insulin, thiazolidinediones, and sulfonylureas. For those who are currently overweight or find it difficult to maintain a healthy weight, this may be difficult. Maintaining a healthy diet, getting more exercise, and seeing a doctor or dietician may all help control the weight gain brought on by these drugs.

4. Fluid Retention: Phoglitazone, a thiazolidinedione, can cause foot and leg edema. People who have cardiac issues may find this especially worrying. Get in touch with your healthcare professional right away if you have severe edema or dyspnea.

5. Genital and Urinary Infections: Because SGLT2 inhibitors raise urine glucose levels, they may increase the risk of vaginal yeast infections and urinary tract infections. This risk may be decreased by practicing excellent hygiene, drinking enough water, and keeping an eye out for signs of illness. Seek immediate medical assistance if you have any symptoms, such as discomfort, burning, or unusual discharge.

Handling medication interactions

Drug interactions may result in more adverse effects or decreased efficacy when one medicine impacts the way another medication functions. People with Type 2 diabetes may be taking many drugs for both diabetes and other medical issues, so managing drug interactions is critical for them.

1. Notify Your Medical Professional of Every Medication: It is important to let your healthcare practitioner know about everything you take, including over-the-counter, prescription, herbal, and supplement medicines. This enables them to monitor for any interactions and modify your treatment plan as necessary.

2. Recognize Typical Interactions: Certain pharmaceuticals and diabetes medicines often interact. For instance, hypoglycemia symptoms may be concealed by certain blood pressure drugs, such as beta-blockers, making it more difficult to identify low blood sugar. Certain drugs, such as corticosteroids, might increase blood sugar, so you may need to modify how you manage your diabetes.

3. Do Not Self-Medicate: Never begin, stop, or alter a medication's dose without first talking to your doctor. This includes nonprescription medicines and dietary supplements, since they may cause interactions with your diabetic treatments. Nonsteroidal anti-inflammatory medicines (NSAIDs), such as ibuprofen, have the potential to impact renal function. This is especially significant for those with

diabetes.

4. Keep an eye out for interactions and side effects: It's critical to regularly check your blood pressure, blood sugar, and general health in order to identify any possible side effects or medication interactions early on. Tell your doctor right away if you have any strange symptoms or changes in your health.

5. Maintain Consistent Contact with Your Healthcare Provider: Scheduling regular follow-up visits with your physician is essential for controlling medication interactions and adverse effects. These consultations allow your doctor to assess your prescriptions, make any necessary changes, and address any concerns.

Diabetes and Cardiovascular Disease

9.1 Understanding the Connection Between Diabetes and Cardiovascular Disease

Heart attacks, strokes, peripheral artery disease, and other cardiovascular disorders (CVD) are all markedly increased by type 2 diabetes. This relationship results from the intricate interactions between insulin resistance, elevated blood sugar, and other metabolic variables that impair heart health and blood vessel integrity.

The process of atherosclerosis, in which fatty deposits (plaque) accumulate and cause the blood vessels to constrict and harden, is one of the main ways diabetes causes cardiovascular problems. High blood sugar levels may harm blood vessel linings, which facilitates the buildup of plaque. Furthermore, diabetes often coexists with other risk factors that exacerbate CVD development, such as high blood pressure, high cholesterol, and obesity.

Controlling Heart Disease

Considering the increased risk, maintaining cardiovascular health is essential to the treatment of diabetes. Here are a few methods to lessen this risk:

Regular Monitoring: It's critical to monitor blood pressure, cholesterol, and sugar levels. Your doctor may advise doing more regular exams to make sure these parameters stay within a healthy range.

Medications: You could be given drugs with the express purpose of decreasing your risk of cardiovascular disease, in addition to drugs that decrease blood sugar. These may include aspirin (to minimize the risk of blood clots), antihypertensives (to control blood pressure), and statins (to lower cholesterol). Always get your doctor's approval before taking any new medications.

Lifestyle Modifications: Reducing the risk of cardiovascular disease may be achieved by implementing a heart-healthy diet, such as the Mediterranean diet, which is high in fruits, vegetables, whole grains, and healthy fats. Frequent exercise, like cycling, swimming, or walking, is also essential for preserving heart health.

Smoking Cessation: Stopping smoking is one of the most important things you can do to protect your heart. The risk of cardiovascular disease is greatly increased by smoking, and it is substantially greater in those with diabetes.

Weight Management: Retaining a healthy weight helps lessen the burden on your heart and lower the possibility of problems. Even a little weight loss may improve the health of your cardiovascular system if you are overweight.

The Significance of Prompt Identification

In its early stages, cardiovascular disease may appear quietly and show little to no symptoms. Early detection and intervention depend on routine tests and check-ups. Chest discomfort, dyspnea, exhaustion, and edema in the legs or feet are symptoms to watch out for. Should you encounter any of these signs, get help right away.

9.2 Diabetic Neuropathy: Damage to Nerves and Pain Control

Diabetic neuropathy: What is it?

A kind of nerve damage known as diabetic neuropathy may develop in diabetics, especially in individuals whose blood sugar levels are inadequately managed over an extended period of time. One of the most common diabetes side effects, it affects 50% of patients. Although neuropathy may affect any area of the body, it often affects the nerves in the feet and legs.

Diabetic neuropathy has a multifactorial etiology, with one of the main culprits being prolonged exposure to elevated blood sugar levels that may harm both the blood vessels that feed the nerve fibers and the sensitive nerves themselves. Inflammation, elevated blood pressure, and high cholesterol are additional contributing factors.

Diabetic Neuropathy Types

Diabetic neuropathy comes in several forms, each with its own unique symptoms and difficulties. They are:

Peripheral Neuropathy: The most prevalent kind of neuropathy first affects the hands and arms before moving on to the feet and legs. Sharp pain, tingling, burning, and numbness are some of the symptoms.

The autonomic nerves, which regulate involuntary bodily activities including digestion, heart rate, and bladder function, are affected by autonomic neuropathy. Urinary tract infections, dizziness, and digestive disorders (such as gastroparesis) are possible symptoms.

Proximal Neuropathy: This kind of neuropathy, often referred to as diabetic amyotrophy, affects the buttocks, thighs, and hips and may result in discomfort, weakness, and muscle atrophy.

Focal Neuropathy: This less common type causes an abrupt loss of strength or discomfort in one or more nerves, usually in the head, chest, or legs.

Controlling pain and neuropathy

Changes in lifestyle, pain management, and blood sugar regulation are all part of managing diabetic neuropathy. The following are some tactics:

Blood Sugar Control: The best strategy to stop or reduce neuropathy development is to maintain strict blood sugar control. Reducing the chance of additional nerve injury may be achieved by maintaining blood glucose levels within the therapeutic range.

drugs for discomfort management: Although neuropathy cannot be cured, drugs may help control discomfort. Prescription drugs, including antidepressants and anticonvulsants, as well as over-the-counter pain medicines and topical remedies like capsaicin cream, are available. Always get your doctor's approval before beginning a new pain management program.

Physical Therapy: By enhancing muscular strength, balance, and coordination, physical therapy may help control symptoms. Certain activities may also help lower discomfort and the chance of falling.

Foot Care: Regular foot care is crucial since neuropathy often affects the feet. This entails cleaning and moisturizing the feet, as well as checking them every day for cuts, blisters, or sores. Another way to reduce the risk of injury is to wear supportive, comfy shoes.

Modifications to Lifestyle: Leading a healthy lifestyle may help control symptoms and enhance general health. This includes controlling stress levels, abstaining from alcohol and tobacco, eating a balanced diet, and getting regular exercise.

When Medical Help Is Needed

It's crucial to speak with your healthcare provider if you suffer from neuropathy symptoms, including continuous numbness, tingling, or discomfort. Prompt care may aid in better symptom management and prevent complications such as infections, foot ulcers, and even amputations.

9.3: Preventing and Treating Kidney Disease

Diabetes and Kidney Disease: A Connection

Diabetic nephropathy, another name for kidney disease, is a dangerous side effect of type 2 diabetes. It happens when the kidneys' small blood vessels are harmed by high blood sugar, making it more difficult for the kidneys to filter waste from the blood. This may eventually result in renal failure or chronic kidney disease (CKD), which may call for dialysis or a kidney transplant.

Diabetes is one of the main causes of chronic kidney disease (CKD), affecting 20–40% of individuals with the condition. The longer someone has diabetes, the higher their chance of developing kidney disease, particularly if they also have high blood pressure, poorly regulated blood sugar, or a family history of kidney disease.

Preventive Techniques
To prevent diabetic kidney disease, diabetes and other risk factors must be managed.

Blood Sugar Control: Maintaining blood sugar levels within the desired range is essential to kidney health. Kidney disease may be delayed or prevented by following your diabetes treatment plan and doing regular monitoring.

Blood Pressure Management: High blood pressure causes renal disease to progress more quickly. Your doctor could advise making lifestyle adjustments, including cutting down on sodium, getting regular exercise, and taking blood pressure medication.

Regular renal function tests: Regular renal function testing may help identify early indicators of kidney disease. These tests include blood tests for creatinine levels and urine tests for albumin, a type of protein. Timely intervention and therapy are made possible by early diagnosis.

Drugs: By decreasing blood pressure and minimizing protein leakage in the urine, some drugs, such as angiotensin-converting enzyme (ACE) inhibitors or angiotensin II receptor blockers (ARBs), are often recommended to protect the kidneys.

Options for Treatment

Treatment for kidney disease focuses on controlling symptoms and reducing the illness's development if it is found:

Dietary Changes: Recommendations for a kidney-friendly diet may include reducing consumption of protein, salt, potassium, and phosphorus. You may manage diabetes and maintain kidney function by developing a food plan in collaboration with a nutritionist.

Medications: Your healthcare practitioner may prescribe drugs to control blood pressure, cholesterol, and blood sugar levels in addition to ACE inhibitors or ARBs. These drugs assist in lessening the kidneys' workload and halting more damage.

Dialysis: When the kidneys are unable to efficiently filter waste in the later stages of renal disease, dialysis may be required. Dialysis is a medical procedure in which the blood is treated using a machine to eliminate waste and extra fluid. Depending on your health and preferences, it may be done at home or at a dialysis clinic.

Kidney Transplant: For some people, a kidney transplant may be an option. This entails surgically replacing the damaged kidney in your body with a healthy kidney from a donor. If organ rejection is avoided, a transplant may provide a higher quality of life than dialysis; nevertheless, immunosuppressive drugs must be used for the rest of one's life.

Living a modified lifestyle, following your treatment plan, and getting frequent checkups from the doctor are all necessary for maintaining kidney health. You may lower your risk of problems and enhance your overall quality of life by managing your diabetes and protecting your kidneys.

9.4: Maintaining Eye Health to Avoid Diabetic Retinopathy

Understanding Retinopathy in Diabetes

Diabetic retinopathy is a common ocular consequence of diabetes. It happens when the small blood vessels in the retina, the light-sensitive layer of tissue at the back of the eye, are harmed by high blood sugar levels. This harm may eventually lead to visual issues, including blindness.

Diabetic retinopathy develops in two primary stages:

Non-Proliferative Diabetic Retinopathy (NPDR): During the first phases, the retina's blood vessels deteriorate and might develop microscopic swellings known as microaneurysms that could leak blood or fluid. This may result in macular edema, or swelling of the retina, which impairs vision.

In more advanced stages, the retina may grow new, brittle blood vessels that are prone to bleeding (proliferative diabetic retinopathy, or PDR). These blood vessels may develop into the vitreous, the gel-like fluid that fills the eye, which may ultimately cause retinal detachment, resulting in significant vision loss, hemorrhage, and scarring.

Early Detection and Prevention

To prevent diabetic retinopathy, diabetes control and routine eye care are required.

Regular eye examinations: To identify diabetic retinopathy in its early stages, yearly, thorough eye examinations are crucial. Throughout the examination, your eye doctor will enlarge your pupils to look for any signs of retinal damage. Early identification enables prompt therapy to stop visual loss.

Blood Sugar Control: Retinopathy cannot proceed as quickly if blood sugar levels are not kept under control. Regular blood sugar monitoring and strict adherence to your diabetes management plan are critical, as elevated blood sugar levels have the potential to worsen the retinal blood vessels.

Control of Blood Pressure and Cholesterol: High blood pressure and cholesterol levels can exacerbate retinopathy. Your eyesight may be protected by controlling these variables with medication and lifestyle modifications.

Healthy Lifestyle: You can maintain eye health and lower your risk of retinopathy by eating a diet high in antioxidants, exercising often, and quitting smoking.

Options for Treatment

Treatment for diabetic retinopathy focuses on protecting eyesight and halting future damage.

Laser Therapy: Abnormal blood vessels in the retina may be sealed or shrunk with laser therapy, sometimes referred to as photocoagulation. This may lessen the chance of eyesight loss and stop more bleeding.

Injections: Anti-VEGF (vascular endothelial growth factor) treatments may help stop the formation of new blood vessels and decrease swelling in the eye. PDR, or macular edema, are two common conditions treated with these injections.

Vitrectomy: To remove blood from the vitreous and heal retinal detachment, an advanced case may need a surgical operation known as a vitrectomy. This process may help to avoid further issues and recover eyesight.

Original Vision Preservation

Maintaining your eyesight demands constant attention and care. By controlling your diabetes, getting regular eye examinations, and acting quickly on any retinopathy symptoms, you can lower your chance of vision loss and preserve the health of your eyes.

9.5 Foot Care: Guarding Against Infections and Ulcers

The Significance of Foot Care in Diabetes

Because Type 2 diabetes increases the risk of nerve damage (neuropathy) and poor circulation, which both raise the risk of foot issues, foot care is an essential part of controlling the disease. Minor foot injuries may necessitate amputation if left untreated and turn into major infections or ulcers.

In addition to slowing down the healing process, diabetic neuropathy may produce numbness in the feet, making it harder to notice injuries. High blood sugar may also weaken the immune system, which raises the risk of infection even more.

Daily Schedule for Foot Care

Keeping your feet healthy and preventing problems may be achieved with a regular regimen of foot care.

Inspect your feet: Every day, look for any irregularities, such as redness, swelling, blisters, wounds, or any sores on your feet. If you need assistance, contact a family member or use a mirror. Severe consequences may be avoided with early issue identification.

Maintain Your Feet Clean: Once a day, use a light soap and warm water to wash your feet. You don't want to bathe your feet because it dries out the skin. To avoid fungal infections, make sure your feet are completely dry, particularly in between the toes.

Moisturize Your Feet: Use a moisturizing lotion to keep your feet's skin supple and protect it from breaking. However, because this region is vulnerable to fungal infections, avoid putting lotion in between the toes.

Trim Toenails Carefully: To avoid ingrown toenails, trim your toenails straight across and file the edges. If you're having trouble cutting your nails, consult a podiatrist for help.

Put on Comfortable Shoes: Opt for shoes that are supportive and fit well. Shoes with pointed toes, high heels, or tight fittings should be avoided since they might create pressure points and result in foot issues. To protect your feet, wear socks with your shoes at all times.

Protect Your Feet: To lower the danger of cuts or injuries, never walk barefoot, even at home. To shield your feet from hot surfaces and sharp objects, put on slippers or shoes.

When Medical Help Is Needed
Seek medical assistance right away if you have any infection-related symptoms, such as redness, swelling, warmth, or pus, or if you have an injury on your foot that doesn't heal in a few days. Minor issues may be stopped before they worsen with early action.

Traditional Foot Care

For specialist foot care, people with diabetes should consult a podiatrist on a regular basis. A podiatrist can expertly care for your nails, remove corns or calluses, and keep an eye out for any indications of potential problems with your feet. Frequent examinations may help avoid foot troubles and guarantee that any that do arise are dealt with right away.

Preserving Your Footwear: In order to effectively manage diabetes, foot care has to be taken care of on a daily basis and examined often. You may lower your risk of ulcers, infections, and other issues, as well as maintain the health and functionality of your feet, by taking proper care of your feet, wearing suitable footwear, and getting medical attention when necessary.

Childhood and Adolescent Diabetes

10.1 The Increasing Rate of Type 2 Diabetes Among Young Individuals

Although type 2 diabetes was long thought to predominantly affect adults, its incidence among children and adolescents has increased considerably in the last several decades. The main causes of this rise include changes in lifestyle, such as poor nutrition, inactivity, and an increase in obesity among younger people.

The emergence of type 2 diabetes in young people raises special concerns, as it may result in a lifetime of health issues, including an increased chance of problems arising early in life. Younger people may also have a more aggressive course of the illness; thus, early identification and treatment are essential.

Identifying the signs

Type 2 diabetes symptoms in kids and teenagers may sometimes be mild and confused with other prevalent illnesses.

Signs to look out for consist of:

Increased Thirst and Urination: Excess glucose from high blood sugar levels leaks into the urine, causing dehydration and increased thirst.
Unexplained Weight Loss: Children with type 2 diabetes may experience weight loss while also having greater hunger because their bodies are unable to use glucose as fuel.
Fatigue: Children may experience chronic fatigue due to a lack of energy, which may make it challenging for them to concentrate in class or remain active.
Blurred Vision: Elevated blood sugar levels may induce fluid to be drawn out of the eye's lenses, impairing vision.
Repeated Infections: Children who have high blood sugar are more vulnerable to infections, especially those of the skin and urinary tract, since it might impair immunity.

Medication and Therapy

For children and adolescents with type 2 diabetes, early diagnosis is crucial to avoiding complications. Usually, many blood tests are used in the diagnosis procedure, including an oral glucose tolerance test, HbA1c, and fasting blood glucose levels.

Young individuals with type 2 diabetes are often treated with a comprehensive strategy that includes lifestyle changes and, sometimes, medication.

Healthy Eating: Maintaining blood sugar levels requires a balanced diet that prioritizes whole grains, fruits, vegetables, lean meats, and healthy fats. It's also critical to cut down on processed meals and sugar-filled beverages.

Regular Physical Activity: Promoting regular exercise, such as riding a bike, walking, or participating in sports, may help regulate weight and enhance insulin sensitivity.

Medication: Healthcare professionals may recommend drugs like metformin, which enhances the body's reaction to insulin, if lifestyle modifications alone are insufficient to regulate blood sugar levels. Insulin treatment could also be required in some circumstances.

Family Involvement: The whole family must take an active role in helping children and adolescents with type 2 diabetes. In order to promote healthy eating, promote physical activity, and guarantee commitment to treatment regimens, parents and other caregivers are essential.

Psychosocial Assistance

For young individuals, having Type 2 diabetes may be physically and psychologically taxing. They could struggle to meet the demands of managing a chronic disease, or they might feel different from their peers. Giving children and teenagers psychological assistance—such as therapy or joining support groups—can help them manage the emotional effects of diabetes and have a positive attitude.

Preventing childhood type 2 diabetes

Promoting good lifestyle choices at a young age is key to preventing type 2 diabetes in children and adolescents. Key tactics include promoting consistent exercise, a nutritious diet, and sustaining a healthy weight. Schools and communities may also help by educating people about healthy living, fostering circumstances that encourage physical exercise, and facilitating access to a diet rich in nutrients.

10.2 Older Adults with Type 2 Diabetes

The Particular Difficulties of Managing Diabetes in the Elderly

Due to population aging, the incidence of type 2 diabetes in the elderly is increasing. The management of diabetes poses distinct difficulties for older persons, such as the coexistence of other chronic ailments, heightened susceptibility to complications, and the possibility of cognitive impairment.

Type 2 diabetes in older people may increase the risk of renal disease, nerve damage, eyesight issues, and cardiovascular disease. Furthermore, reduced mobility, sensory abnormalities, and polypharmacy (the use of numerous drugs) could complicate diabetes treatment in this group.

Determining Personalized Therapy Objectives

Treatment plans for older people with Type 2 diabetes should be tailored to each patient's health status, life expectancy, and co-existing chronic illnesses. In order to lower the risk of hypoglycemia, or low blood sugar, which may be especially harmful in this demographic, older people's objectives may be more flexible than those of younger people.

Blood Sugar Targets: An HbA1c goal level of less than 7.5% may be suitable for healthy older people with few additional medical concerns. To reduce the risk of hypoglycemia, a goal of less than 8–8.5% may be more appropriate for those with numerous chronic illnesses or a short life expectancy.

Blood Pressure and Cholesterol Management: Reducing the risk of cardiovascular disease still requires careful monitoring of blood pressure and cholesterol levels. Nonetheless, the course of therapy should take the patient's general health and any possible drug adverse effects into account.

Weight Management: While maintaining a healthy weight is crucial, reaching a particular weight goal should not take precedence over general well-being and quality of life. While inadvertent weight loss in the elderly should be looked into, minor weight reduction may sometimes enhance diabetes control.

Medicine Administration

In order to treat a variety of medical ailments, older people are often given many drugs, which raises the possibility of drug interactions and adverse consequences. Healthcare professionals should carefully examine drug selection while treating diabetes in the elderly, with the goal of reducing the risk of hypoglycemia and associated side effects.

Streamlining Treatment Regimens: Whenever feasible, streamlining the drug schedule may ease the strain on senior patients and enhance compliance. This may include taking drugs like metformin or DPP-4 inhibitors, which have a decreased risk of hypoglycemia.

Side Effects Monitoring: Seniors are more vulnerable to drug side effects; thus, frequent monitoring is crucial. This includes monitoring renal function, hypoglycemic symptoms, and any medication interactions.

Deprescribing: If a medicine's hazards exceed its benefits, it may be reasonable to reduce or stop prescribing it in certain circumstances. The healthcare provider should be consulted before making this choice.

Tackling Diabetes and Cognitive Decline

Older people with type 2 diabetes are more likely to have cognitive deterioration, including dementia. Individuals with cognitive impairment may need extra assistance in managing their diabetes because they may have trouble remembering to take their prescriptions, adhering to dietary recommendations, or identifying hypoglycemic symptoms.

Support Systems: Ensuring that an aged person receiving optimal diabetic care is made easier by establishing a support system including family members, caretakers, or home health aides. Assistance with drug management and regular check-ins might be helpful.

Routine Screening: Elderly people with diabetes may benefit from routine cognitive screening to spot early indicators of cognitive loss. Early identification enables diabetes care to be modified to take the person's cognitive skills into account.

Encouraging Life Quality

Encouraging an excellent quality of life is the ultimate aim of diabetes treatment for the elderly. This entails preserving autonomy, averting issues, and promoting mental and physical health. For older people with diabetes, a balanced diet, social interaction, and regular physical exercise are essential elements of a healthy lifestyle.

10.3: Handling Gestational Diabetes During Pregnancy

Understanding Diabetes During Pregnancy

One kind of diabetes that affects how the body uses glucose during pregnancy is called gestational diabetes. It generally appears during the second or third trimester of pregnancy and goes away after delivery. On the other hand, women who acquire gestational diabetes have a higher chance of acquiring type 2 diabetes in the future.

When the body cannot make enough insulin to fulfill the increasing needs of pregnancy, gestational diabetes results. This leads to higher blood sugar levels, which may be dangerous for the mother and the unborn child. Being overweight, having a family history of diabetes, being older than 25, and being a member of certain ethnic groups are risk factors for gestational diabetes.

Diagnosis and Screening

It is customary to screen for gestational diabetes between weeks 24 and 28 of pregnancy. The oral glucose tolerance test (OGTT), which gauges the body's reaction to glucose, is the most widely used screening technique.

Early management is essential to controlling blood sugar

levels and lowering the risk of complications if gestational diabetes is confirmed. This might include altering one's lifestyle, checking one's blood sugar, and sometimes taking medicine.

Controlling Diabetes During Pregnancy

To maintain blood sugar levels within a target range, managing gestational diabetes entails a mix of lifestyle changes and, if required, medication.

Healthy Eating: Managing gestational diabetes requires a balanced diet. Make sure you eat enough fruits, veggies, whole grains, lean meats, and healthy fats. In order to minimize blood sugar spikes, it's also critical to keep an eye on your carbohydrate consumption and spread it evenly throughout the day.

Regular Physical Activity: Exercise lowers blood sugar and increases insulin sensitivity. Pregnant women may safely participate in most activities, including walking, swimming, and prenatal yoga, but it's crucial to speak with your doctor before beginning any fitness regimen.

Blood Sugar Monitoring: In order to effectively manage gestational diabetes, blood sugar levels must be regularly monitored. You may follow your healthcare provider's instructions on how often to check your levels and what range to strive for.

Medication: Your healthcare practitioner may recommend

insulin or other safe-to-use drugs if lifestyle modifications alone are insufficient to regulate blood sugar levels. It's important to heed the advice of your healthcare practitioner and modify your treatment plan as necessary.

Surveillance and Provision

Preterm birth, excessive birth weight (macrosomia), and the requirement for a cesarean delivery are among the pregnancy and delivery issues that are more likely to occur in women with gestational diabetes.

To guarantee the health of the mother and the unborn child, routine prenatal examinations and monitoring are crucial.

Fetal Monitoring: To track the baby's growth and development, routine ultrasound examinations may be carried out. Additionally, your doctor will check your urine and blood pressure for indications of preeclampsia, a disease that may occur in pregnant women with gestational diabetes.

Delivery Plan: To reduce the chance of difficulties, your healthcare practitioner will collaborate with you to create a delivery plan. If the baby is big or if there are additional concerns, it may be advised in certain situations to deliver the infant early.

Care After Giving Birth

Gestational diabetes normally goes away after giving birth, but in the weeks that follow, it's crucial to keep an eye on your blood sugar levels. Long-term health depends on regular checkups and lifestyle changes, since women with gestational diabetes are more likely to acquire Type 2 diabetes.

Breastfeeding: Breastfeeding reduces the risk of developing type 2 diabetes and is good for both the mother and the child. Additionally, it aids in postpartum weight reduction, which is crucial for controlling the risk of diabetes.

frequent Screening: In order to keep an eye out for the onset of Type 2 diabetes, women who have had gestational diabetes should undergo frequent diabetes tests, as advised by their healthcare professional.

10.4 Diabetes and Mental Health: Taking Care of Anxiety and Depression

The Relationship Between Mental Health and Diabetes

Diabetes type 2 may have a negative impact on mental health, increasing the risk of disorders including anxiety and depression. Emotional discomfort may be exacerbated by the ongoing care of the illness, worry about future consequences, and the effect on day-to-day living. Furthermore, mood and mental health may be impacted by the physiological impacts of diabetes, such as changes in blood sugar levels.

Studies have shown that there is a higher likelihood of anxiety and depression in those with diabetes compared to people without the illness. On the other hand, anxiety and depression may make it harder to successfully control diabetes, which can lead to a vicious cycle of stress and adverse health consequences.

Identifying the Signs of Anxiety and Depression

Diabetes patients may exhibit symptoms of worry and sadness, which should be recognized as early treatment may enhance both physical and emotional well-being. Symptoms of depression may include:

Extended depressive or despairing sentiments
A decline in interest in formerly cherished hobbies
Lethargy or lack of energy
Having trouble focusing or coming to conclusions
Alterations to eating or sleeping habits
Suicidal or self-harming thoughts

Anxiety symptoms might include:

Overwhelming anxiety or terror, anxiety or a restless sensation -Sensitivity, Tension in the muscles, disturbances in sleep, episodes of panic

It's critical to get medical attention from a professional if you or someone you know is experiencing these symptoms.

The Effect of Mental Health on the Management of Diabetes

Effective diabetes management may be more challenging for those with mental health issues. Poor self-care practices, such as skipping blood sugar checks, adopting bad food habits, and engaging in less physical exercise, may be brought on by depression and anxiety. These actions may thus exacerbate diabetes management and raise the possibility of complications.

On the other hand, proper diabetes management may benefit mental health. Maintaining a nutritious diet, getting regular exercise, and controlling blood sugar levels may all help elevate mood and lessen the signs of anxiety and sadness.

Management Techniques for Mental Health in Diabetes

Addressing mental health is an essential part of providing comprehensive diabetes treatment. The following are some methods to promote mental health:

Seek professional support: You should think about getting assistance from a mental health professional if you are exhibiting signs of anxiety or sadness. Therapy, including cognitive-behavioral therapy (CBT), is useful for enhancing coping mechanisms and correcting maladaptive thinking patterns.

Medication: Prescription drugs may sometimes be recommended to treat anxiety or depression. It's crucial to talk to your healthcare practitioner about any possible interactions between your diabetic medicines.

Mindfulness and Stress Reduction: Activities that promote mindfulness, including yoga, deep breathing, and meditation, may reduce stress and enhance mental clarity. Including these routines in your everyday life may improve your general health.

Social Support: Making connections with others who are aware of the difficulties associated with having diabetes may lessen feelings of loneliness and provide emotional support. To exchange stories and get help, think about joining a support group or participating in online communities.

Healthy Lifestyle: You may improve your physical and mental well-being by leading a healthy lifestyle that includes frequent exercise, a balanced diet, and enough sleep. Exercise, in particular, has been shown to elevate mood and lessen signs of anxiety and despair.

The Function of Medical Professionals

When it comes to meeting the mental health needs of people with diabetes, healthcare professionals are essential. An integral component of diabetes management should include periodic screening for anxiety and depression. In addition, providers may provide resources for stress management and coping mechanisms, as well as connections to mental health specialists.

Taking care of your mental health is equally as important as regulating your blood sugar levels while managing diabetes. Understanding the link between diabetes and mental health, getting help from a professional, and using beneficial coping mechanisms may all help you live a better life and manage your diabetes more skillfully.

Lifestyle Interventions to Prevent Type 2 Diabetes

11.1 Be aware of how lifestyle affects type 2 diabetes prevention

Because lifestyle choices have an enormous influence on lowering the chance of developing type 2 diabetes, the illness is usually avoidable. Making healthy dietary and lifestyle choices can significantly reduce your risk of getting Type 2 diabetes, even if genetics and other uncontrollable variables still play a role.

Nutritious Eating Practices

Following a nutritious diet that promotes stable blood sugar levels and a healthy weight is one of the best strategies to avoid type 2 diabetes. Here are some essential eating techniques:

Highlight whole foods: Place an emphasis on consuming unprocessed, whole foods, including fruits, vegetables, whole grains, lean meats, and healthy fats. These meals support blood sugar regulation and provide vital nutrients.

Control Portion Sizes: Consuming large amounts of even healthful meals might lead to weight gain. Limiting portion sizes may help to manage calorie intake and prevent overindulgence in food.

Select complex carbs: Since complex carbs are absorbed more slowly, they cause blood sugar levels to rise gradually. Examples of these include whole grains, legumes, and vegetables. Sugary meals and processed carbs should be avoided because they can quickly raise blood sugar levels.

Increase Fiber Intake: Foods rich in fiber, such as fruits, vegetables, whole grains, and legumes, help control blood sugar levels by delaying sugar absorption. In addition to promoting fullness, fiber also helps regulate appetite and prevent overeating.

Reduce sugary drinks: Sugary beverages, such as fruit juice, soda, and energy drinks, may cause sharp swings in blood sugar levels and cause weight gain. Choose drinks with minimal or no added sugar, herbal teas, or water.

Daily Exercise

Including regular exercise in your daily routine is another effective way to stave off type 2 diabetes. Exercise increases insulin sensitivity, allowing your body to use glucose more efficiently. Here's how to include exercise in your daily routine:

Aim for Consistency: The objective is to do 150 minutes or more of moderate-intensity aerobic exercise, such as swimming, cycling, or brisk walking, each week. If you find this intimidating, begin with shorter sessions and progressively extend them.

Incorporate Strength Training: Activities that increase muscle mass, such as lifting weights or using resistance bands, improve your body's capacity to use insulin. Aim for two or more sessions of strength training per week.

Remain active throughout the day: Aim to remain active throughout the day in addition to scheduled exercise. This may be achieved by going for quick walks, getting up regularly from sedentary work, and opting for active transportation choices like bicycling or walking rather than driving.

Find Activities You Enjoy: Long-term enjoyment and commitment to an exercise regimen are the keys to optimal fitness. Whether it's yoga, hiking, dancing, or participating in sports, find physical activities that you like and include them in your daily routine.

Control of Weight

Remaining within a healthy weight range is essential for avoiding type 2 diabetes. Being overweight raises insulin resistance and the chance of acquiring diabetes, especially around the belly. The following are some methods for reaching and maintaining a healthy weight:

Set realistic goals: Put more effort into making little, long-lasting lifestyle improvements than you would into rapidly losing weight. It is possible to greatly reduce your chance of developing Type 2 diabetes by aiming to lose 5–10% of your body weight.

Monitor Your Progress: To remain accountable and make necessary modifications, keep a record of your food consumption, amount of exercise, and weight. By self-monitoring on a regular basis, you can remain on course and acknowledge little accomplishments along the way.

Seek Support: Take into account collaborating with a trained dietician, attending a weight reduction group, or asking friends and family for help. Having a solid support network may keep you motivated and enable you to overcome obstacles.

Reducing alcohol intake

Overindulging in alcohol may increase the risk of developing type 2 diabetes and lead to weight gain. If you decide to consume alcohol, do so sparingly. This translates to a maximum of one drink for women and a maximum of two for men every day. When selecting an alcoholic beverage, keep in mind that some types have more calories than others.

Stress Reduction

Persistent stress may harm your health and raise your chance of getting type 2 diabetes. Diabetes develops as a result of harmful habits like smoking, overeating, and skipping exercise that are brought on by stress. Reducing stress and promoting a healthy lifestyle may be achieved by putting stress management strategies like yoga, deep breathing exercises, and mindfulness meditation into practice.

11.2 Stress Reduction and Blood Sugar Effects

Understanding the Relationship Between Blood Sugar and Stress

Although stress is a normal part of life, it may negatively affect your physical health if it persists for an extended period of time, especially if you have Type 2 diabetes or are at risk for it. Hormones like cortisol and adrenaline are released while under stress, preparing your body for a "fight or flight" reaction. As a result of these hormones' increased hepatic glucose release into the blood, blood glucose levels may rise.

Chronic stress may make it more difficult for people with type 2 diabetes to control their blood sugar levels, resulting in swings that can exacerbate symptoms. Stress can also lead to bad habits such as binge eating, inactivity, and restless nights, all of which can worsen the illness.

Signs of Stress Recognition

In order to properly manage stress, it's essential to identify its telltale signals. Typical stress indicators include:

Emotional Symptoms: agitation, mood fluctuations, anxiety, and depressive or overwhelming sensations.
Physical symptoms include headaches, tense muscles, exhaustion, and digestive problems.

Behavioral Symptoms: alterations in appetite, insomnia, disorganization, and social disengagement.

If any of these symptoms apply to you, stress-reduction techniques may help improve your health.

Strategies for Stress Management
Effective stress management strategies include the following, many of which may help improve blood sugar regulation and general wellbeing:

Mindfulness and Meditation: By increasing your awareness of your thoughts and emotions, mindfulness meditation may help you react to stress in a more composed manner. Frequent meditation has been shown to enhance blood sugar levels, decrease blood pressure, and reduce stress.

Physical Activity: Physical activity helps reduce cortisol levels and elevate mood. It's a natural stress reliever. Exercises that assist blood sugar regulation and relieve stress include yoga, running, walking, and swimming.

Deep Breathing Exercises: By triggering the body's relaxation response, deep breathing exercises like diaphragmatic breathing may lower tension and foster a feeling of serenity. To help reduce stress, spend a few minutes each day practicing deep breathing.

Progressive Muscle Relaxation: This method may help relieve physical tension and lower stress by first tensing and then relaxing various muscle groups in the body.

Social Support: Making connections with loved ones, friends, or support groups may help you manage stress and provide emotional support. Speaking with a trusted person about your emotions might reduce stress and provide new insight.

Time Management: Stress and overload may result from ineffective time management. Delegating duties, setting reasonable objectives, and prioritizing work are all skills that may lower stress and boost output.

Including Stress Reduction in Your Everyday Activities

It's critical to include stress management into your everyday routine in order to properly manage stress and its effects on blood sugar. Here are some pointers:

Begin your day with relaxation: To create a pleasant tone for the day, start your morning with a few minutes of deep breathing, meditation, or gentle stretching.

Take Regular Breaks: Take quick pauses throughout the day to unwind and refuel. Stress may be reduced, even for a short while, with deep breathing exercises or a fast stroll.

Eat With Awareness: Eating with awareness may help you choose better foods and avoid emotional eating, which is often brought on by stress. Savor every mouthful and pay heed to your body's signals of hunger and fullness.

Completing Your Day with Relaxation: Unwind at night with a soothing pastime like light yoga, reading, or a warm bath. This may help you decompress and prepare for a good night's sleep.

The Extended Advantages of Stress Reduction

Regular stress management lowers the risk of diabetes-related problems and promotes improved blood sugar regulation, in addition to improving your mental and emotional health. By incorporating stress management practices into your daily routine, you can raise your standard of living and improve your overall health.

11.3 Sleep's Significance in Diabetes Care

The Significance of Good Sleep

Sleep, a vital component of overall health and wellbeing, is essential for blood sugar management and metabolic stability. Lack of sleep may significantly affect blood sugar levels and diabetes management.

Research has shown a link between poor sleep quality, sleep deprivation, elevated insulin resistance, elevated blood sugar, and an increased risk of type 2 diabetes. Furthermore, a lack of sleep may worsen diabetes by causing weight gain, increased hunger, and unwise dietary choices.

The Effect of Lack of Sleep on Blood Sugar

Your body produces more cortisol, a stress hormone that elevates blood sugar, when you don't get enough sleep. In addition, a lack of sleep might lower insulin sensitivity, which can complicate your body's ability to use glucose. The confluence of these variables may result in elevated blood glucose levels and complicate diabetes treatment.

Moreover, the absence of hormones that control hunger and

fullness may be upset by sleep deprivation, which can increase appetite and cause cravings for high-calorie, sugary meals. This may worsen blood sugar regulation and lead to weight gain.

Guides for Enhancing the Quality of Sleep

Enhancing the quality of your sleep may benefit your general health and blood sugar levels. Here are some pointers to help you sleep better:

Create a Regular Sleep Schedule: Every day, even on the weekends, I go to bed and wake up at the same time. This improves sleep quality by balancing your body's natural clock.

Establish a Calm Bedtime Routine: Establish a peaceful bedtime ritual that tells your body it's time to unwind. This might include doing things like reading, taking a warm bath, or using deep breathing techniques.

Create a Comfortable Sleep Environment: Make sure your bedroom is quiet, dark, and cool to sleep in. To encourage sound sleep, spend money on pillows and a quality mattress.

Reduce Alcohol and Caffeine: Alcohol and caffeine may both affect the quality of your sleep. Aim to stay away from these things in the hours before going to bed.

Reduce Screen Time Before Bed: Your body's melatonin production, which controls sleep, may be disrupted by the blue light produced by phones, tablets, and laptops. Try to switch off devices an hour or more before going to bed.

Remain Active During the Day: Getting regular exercise can help you sleep deeper and fall asleep more quickly. Avoid engaging in strenuous activity too soon before bed, however, since this might have a stimulating impact.

Control tension: Prolonged tension might lower the quality of your sleep. You may unwind and get a better night's sleep by incorporating stress-reduction methods into your daily routine, such as progressive muscle relaxation or mindfulness meditation.

The Relationship Between Sleep and Controlling Your Weight

Sleep quality has a direct impact on weight management, which is critical for both preventing and treating type 2 diabetes. You're more likely to maintain a healthy weight, choose healthier foods, and have more energy for physical exercise when you get enough sleep. On the other hand, insufficient sleep may result in increased insulin resistance, weight gain, and elevated blood sugar.

Seeking assistance for sleep issues

You should consult a healthcare professional if you're experiencing sleep issues, including insomnia, sleep apnea, or restless legs syndrome. Resolving sleep problems may help you manage your diabetes better and have a higher quality of life overall.

11.4 Diabetes and Quitting Smoking

Smoking's Hazards for Individuals with Diabetes
In addition to being one of the biggest risk factors for type 2 diabetes, smoking may exacerbate the disease's consequences for those who already have it. Compared to non-smokers, smokers have a 30–40% increased risk of Type 2 diabetes, and this risk rises with cigarette use.

 Smoking may result in a number of dangerous health issues for diabetics, such as:

Increased Insulin Resistance: Nicotine from cigarettes may lead to an increase in insulin resistance, which will hinder your body's ability to use glucose as efficiently as possible. This may result in elevated blood glucose levels and complicate the treatment of diabetes.

Cardiovascular Complications: Smoking exacerbates the risk of cardiovascular disease, which is already higher in people with diabetes, by damaging blood vessels. Diabetes increases the risk of heart attacks, strokes, and other cardiovascular problems among smokers.

Increased Risk of Issues: Renal disease, neuropathy, and retinopathy are among the diabetes-related issues that smoking may aggravate. Additionally, it slows down the healing process, which raises the possibility of infections and ulcers, especially on the foot.

Worsened Lung Health: Smoking may cause lung diseases such as chronic obstructive pulmonary disease (COPD), which can make managing diabetes more difficult and lower the quality of life overall.

The benefits of quitting smoking

One of the best things you can do for your health is to stop smoking, especially if you have diabetes. Among the advantages of quitting smoking are:

Improved Insulin Sensitivity: Giving up smoking will help your body become more insulin-sensitive, which will help you regulate your blood sugar levels.

Decreased chance of cardiovascular disease: Giving up smoking lowers your chance of heart disease, stroke, and other cardiovascular-related issues dramatically. The chance of having a heart attack dramatically decreases after a year of stopping.

Lowered Risk of Complications: Giving up smoking may lower your chance of developing diabetes-related problems such as neuropathy, retinopathy, and kidney disease. Additionally, it increases circulation, which facilitates faster healing and lowers the risk of infections and ulcers.

Better lung health: Giving up smoking may enhance your

general health and quality of life by improving lung function and lowering your chance of developing chronic respiratory disorders.

Techniques for smoking cessation

Although quitting smoking might be difficult, it is possible with the correct techniques and assistance. The following advice will help you stop smoking:

Set a Quit Date: Decide on a definite day to give up smoking and be ready, both physically and psychologically. In order for them to support you, let your friends, family, and healthcare provider know about your plan.

Use Nicotine Replacement Therapy (NRT): Products that substitute nicotine, including gum, lozenges, patches, or inhalers, might lessen cravings and withdrawal symptoms. What is the best NRT choice for you? Discuss this with your healthcare practitioner.

Look into prescription medications: Prescription drugs are available to help lessen withdrawal symptoms and cravings. It is important to use these drugs under a doctor's supervision.

Identify triggers: Note the events, feelings, or pursuits that set off your desire for smoke. Create coping mechanisms to deal with or prevent these triggers, such as deep breathing exercises, walks, or stress balls.

Seek Support: To connect with others who are attempting to stop smoking, think about enrolling in a support group or program. The psychological components of addiction may also be effectively addressed with the aid of behavioral treatment and counseling.

Remain Upbeat: Giving up smoking is a journey, and obstacles are common along the way. Remind yourself of the health advantages of quitting smoking, maintain your positive attitude, and concentrate on your reasons for doing so.

The Function of Medical Professionals

You may get important support from your healthcare provider to help you stop smoking. They may provide you with direction, materials, and encouragement to help you achieve. Keeping track of your progress and addressing any obstacles you may have along the way may be accomplished with regular follow-up sessions.

Lifestyle Decisions Are Critical for Diabetes Management

A multimodal strategy that incorporates stress management, physical exercise on a regular basis, a healthy diet, proper sleep hygiene, and quitting smoking is necessary to prevent and treat type 2 diabetes. By adopting healthy lifestyle choices, you can significantly lower your risk of diabetes, improve blood sugar management, and improve your overall quality of life.